Praise for *Thrive Foods*

"Drawing from studies preformed by top international organizations, Brendan Brazier cuts through the clutter. Putting the information into clear and relatable terms, he effectively illustrates the easiest, most immediate, and most dramatic form of activism we can all participate in: choosing our food. *Thrive Foods* is the definitive guide to nourishing ourselves, while deliciously saving our world. It's time to Thrive!"
—Elizabeth J. Kucinich, director of public and government affairs, Physicians Committee for Responsible Medicine

"*Thrive Foods* makes the art of healthy eating and the concept of a nutrient dense diet easy to understand and compelling to follow. A must read for anyone who wants to be healthy, live longer, and eat the best foods our planet has to offer."
—Terry Tamminen, former chief policy advisor to Governor Schwarzenegger, president of Seventh Generation Advisors

"The world needs to move away from meat. As Brendan Brazier so convincingly shows, a plant-based diet is better for the planet and better for human health. His wonderfully inventive vegan recipes give us food that is both nutritious and inviting."
—Chris Goodall, bestselling author of *How to Live a Low Carbon Life*

"Brendan Brazier has helped top athletes achieve a whole new level of performance through optimal nutrition, and now he's helping readers everywhere reach peak health. Brendan Brazier is your guide to getting healthy and fit through optimal nutrition. I have long relied on Brendan's expertise, and you will, too. And the recipes are almost as fast as Brendan is! Each one is quick, easy, and delicious, so you'll be off and running in no time!"
—Neal Barnard, M.D., president, Physicians Committee for Responsible Medicine

Praise for *Thrive* and *Thrive Fitness*

"Brendan's knowledge is second to none."
—Simon Whitfield, Olympic gold medalist
(triathlon, Sydney 2000)

"*Thrive* is an eye-opening and a life-changing book.
It should replace bibles in hotels."
—Dave Zabriskie, professional cyclist,
Tour de France stage winner, and record holder of the
fastest time trial in Tour de France history

"*Thrive* has revolutionized the way I go about fueling my
body and helped push me to a higher level of performance and
workout recovery. There's no other resource like it out there."
—Mac Danzig, Ultimate Fighter 6 champion

"*Thrive* is a life-changing book!"
—Jon Hinds, former LA Clippers strength-training coach
and advisor to MLB and NFL teams

"*Thrive* is an authoritative guide to outstanding performance,
not just in top-level athletics but in day-to-day life."
—Neal D. Barnard, M.D., president,
Physicians Committee for Responsible Medicine

"Brendan Brazier's *Thrive* will increase the micronutrient density of your
eating style and enable you to live longer, live healthier, and thrive."
—Joel Fuhrman, M.D., bestselling author of *Eat to Live* and *Eat for Health*

"*Thrive* is a must read."
—T. Colin Campbell, Ph.D., author of the bestselling *The China Study*

"Quite possibly the most life-changing book you'll ever read.
For maximizing fitness and vitality, *Thrive* has no equal."
—Erik Marcus, publisher of Vegan.com

"Quite simply, *Thrive* is the most comprehensive nutrition
and lifestyle program we've ever seen."
—The G Living Network

THRIVE FOODS

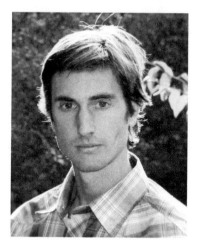

A former professional Ironman triathlete, and a two-time Canadian 50 km Ultra Marathon champion, BRENDAN BRAZIER is the author of *Thrive* and *Thrive Fitness*, as well as the creator of an award-winning line of whole food nutritional products called Vega.

Recognized as one of the world's foremost authorities on plant-based nutrition, Brendan is a guest lecturer at Cornell University and presents an eCornell module entitled "The Plant-Based Diet and Elite Athleticism."

Brendan was chosen as one of the 25 Most Fascinating Vegetarians by *VegNews Magazine* and named one of the Top 40 Under 40 most influential people in the health industry by Natural Food Merchandiser. He has been nominated three times for the prestigious Manning Innovation Award for the creation of the Vega formula.

brendanbrazier.com

Also by **Brendan Brazier**

Thrive Fitness

Thrive

THRIVE FOODS

200 PLANT-BASED
RECIPES FOR PEAK HEALTH

BRENDAN BRAZIER

Da Capo
LIFE
LONG

A Member of the Perseus Books Group

Graphics created by Tommy Heiden

Cataloging-in-Publication data for this book is available from the Library of Congress.

First Da Capo Press edition 2011
Thrive Foods: 200 Plant-Based Recipes for Peak Health was originally published in 2011 by the Penguin Group (Canada) as *Whole Foods to Thrive: Nutrient-Dense, Plant-Based Recipes for Peak Health*. This edition is published by arrangement with the Penguin Group (Canada).
PB ISBN: 978-0-7382-1511-2
E-book ISBN: 978-0-7382-1512-9
Library of Congress Control Number: 2011928480

Published by Da Capo Press
A Member of the Perseus Books Group
www.dacapopress.com

Da Capo Press books are available at special discounts for bulk purchases in the U.S. by corporations, institutions, and other organizations. For more information, please contact the Special Markets Department at the Perseus Books Group, 2300 Chestnut Street, Suite 200, Philadelphia, PA, 19103, or call (800) 810-4145, ext. 5000, or e-mail special.markets@perseusbooks.com.

10 9

CONTENTS

DRINKS

BREAKFASTS

SALADS

SOUPS AND SIDES

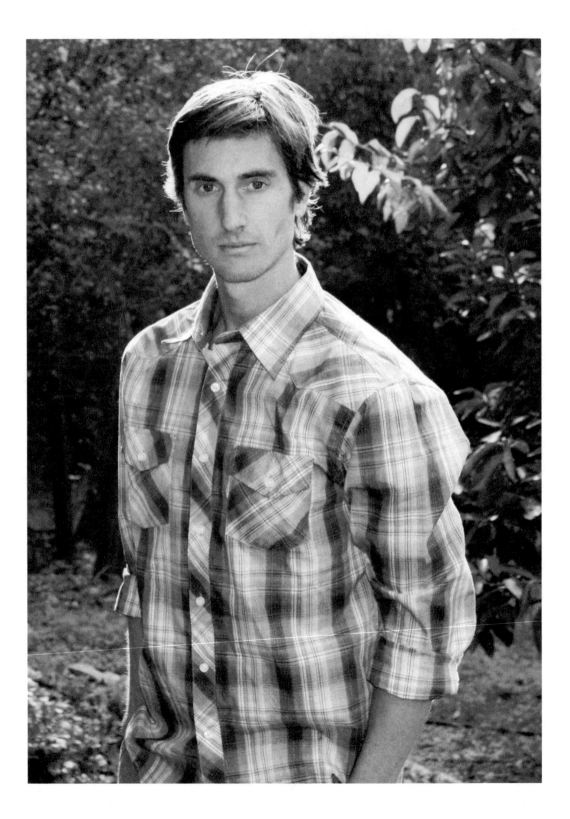

INTRODUCTION

Coming from an athletic background, I developed my interest in food simply as a means for enhancing performance. I wanted the best fuel and biological building blocks available. But after several years of being meticulous about what I ate, it dawned on me that I actually knew very little about food itself. While I understood nutrition—the components that make up food—I knew very little about food as a whole: where it came from, who grew it, how much time needed to pass for it to go from seed to ready-to-eat food, etc. And how did my food choices affect all those involved along the way? Then there were the environmental considerations. What was the environmental draw of the laborious process of converting natural resources into edible sustenance?

When I selected what to eat, I understood that choice most certainly had a direct impact on health and performance (which I discuss in Chapter 1), but I was only just beginning to appreciate the broad and significant influence that our individual food choices have on the lives of others and how our food choices impact the environment.

The significance of this began to sink in, and as it did, an appreciation for the scope of influence our food choices had—one that extended far beyond us as individuals—came with it.

In fact, it's that appreciation that led me to write this book. While my interest in food had been sparked by a selfish desire for premium nutrition to fuel athletic performance, as I pried deeper into the world of food, I became fascinated with the system as a whole.

I began asking questions.

Undeniably, unrefined whole food is an essential component to good health, but what attribute determines a food's nutritional quality? Caloric density? Vitamins? Minerals? Phytochemicals? Antioxidants? I wanted to know. And what is the environmental cost of each of these nutritional components? Certainly not all foods are equal in their nutritional makeup, but how do each of their impacts on the environment compare?

I wrote this book in pursuit of those answers. What I found fascinated me. The choices each of us makes every day as to what we'll eat turned out to have a greater impact than I ever could have imagined.

Starting off with a focus on obtaining peak health, I begin by discussing a North American epidemic, one of the leading causes of disease and unrealized potential: stress. The subject of my first book, *Thrive*, stress has become a ubiquitous part of our modern lives. Unfortunately, its familiar symptoms—difficulty sleeping, inability to lose body fat despite regular exercise, sugar and starch cravings, dependence on stimulants such as coffee to start the day, and general fatigue hitting around two o'clock in the afternoon—have become the rule, not the exception. Depending on its nutritional makeup, food can either contribute to or help alleviate overall stress.

I examine what nutritional characteristics to consider when making food choices to better nourish the body, and therefore to reduce stress through the consumption of higher quality food.

As I found, micronutrient content, known as nutrient density, is the most comprehensive measure of the health-boosting properties of a given food. The greater the nutrient density, the less nutritional stress (the biological strain created when nutritional requirements are not adequately met). I give a detailed account of nutritional stress in Chapter 1.

In addition to advocating that your first consideration in choosing food should be its nutrient density, I propose a set of "guiding principles" to use when selecting what to eat.

In Chapter 2, I look at the environmental toll levied in the food-production process. Our health is, overwhelmingly, tied to the quality of the food we eat. And food quality is directly tied to the quality of the soil in which it was grown. Therefore, the health of the environment has a direct tie to our health by way of food (not to mention by way of the air we breathe and the water we drink).

> Growing and processing food not only consume land, water, and fossil fuel but also create carbon emissions.

Since plants pull minerals from the soils—micronutrients essential for human health—they serve as a conduit, taking the soil—the environment—putting it into a digestible form, and passing it on to us. Each time we take a bite of food, part of the environment literally becomes part of our biological fabric, our bodies. At the risk of sounding like a hippy, the Earth is part of us.

This being the case—if for no other reason than personal self-interest—it's worthwhile taking environmental preservation measures. But there are larger reasons for caring about food. In return for food, we exchange a considerable amount of natural resources. Growing and processing food not only consume land, water, and fossil fuel but also create carbon emissions.

In Chapter 3, I examine what others have done to address the vast global environmental strain of food production. The U.K. government leads the way in offering carbon labels on food to give consumers some perspective as to the effect their food choices have on carbon emissions production, and therefore on environmental health. I also explore steps progressive companies, such as Whole Foods Markets, are taking to help consumers make healthy choices by indicating the nutrient density of many of their food items.

Having had the opportunity to work with some of the best minds in the nutrition world, as well as with some leading environmental advocates, I have developed an appreciation of two different perspectives, which haven't often converged.

In being exposed to the connection between personal and environmental health, I dedicate a large part of Chapter 3 to the marriage of the two. I call this connection the "nutrient-to-resource ratio."

I also examine the monetary cost of food. Undoubtedly it's less expensive to gain calories from highly processed food. But what about micronutrients—the true measure of food value—what's the least expensive way to obtain them? I explore this question, displaying my findings by using icons that clearly display the good from the less desirable.

Rounding out the chapter, I visually showcase the environmental strain involved in producing a day of meals following, first, a Standard American Diet, and next following what is commonly perceived as a

"Healthy" American diet. Finally, I look at the environmental strain of producing a day's meal plan using the whole foods recipes in this book. The contrast was sharper than I could have imagined.

In Chapter 4, I go on to consider eight key nutritional components, and their benefits, that are worth seeking when making food choices.

In Chapter 5, I suggest specific foods that have health-boosting and environmental-preserving attributes described earlier in the book. The section "Whole Foods to Thrive Pantry Essentials" provides a list of staples that will help you keep your kitchen well stocked with the essential ingredients for whole food meals.

The book culminates with 200 fabulous recipes, all made with nutrient-dense, plant-based whole foods that are both health-boosting and easy on the environment.

Created with help from some top chef friends, all the recipes in this final chapter adhere to my nutritional philosophy.

Feature Chefs

While I created all the recipes in both *Thrive* and *Thrive Fitness*, as well as some of the recipes in this book, I grew curious as to how top-tier chefs would approach recipe creation using nutrient-dense, plant-based whole food ingredients.

And, since I'm by no means a chef, I felt there must certainly be flavor profiles and ingredient combinations—unknown to me—that would increase palatability and overall appeal. For this reason, I enlisted the help of a few of my favorite chefs.

The chef creating most of the recipes—about half of the book's total—is Julie Morris. Julie is a Los Angeles–based natural food chef who has the unique ability to draw and balance a wide range of flavors from natural whole foods ingredients.

> All the recipes are nutrient-dense, tread lightly on the environment, and taste amazing.

In keeping with the nutritional philosophy of this book, Julie has taken a truly novel and creative approach in developing delicious, accessible, and easy-to-make recipes out of premium, nutrient-dense, health-boosting ingredients.

The other top chefs I've enlisted have each contributed two to four world-class, plant-based, whole food creations, all of which, I think you'll agree, are truly delicious.

All the recipes here are nutrient-dense, tread lightly on the environment, and taste amazing. One of the most pleasing aspects of these recipes is their diversity. From simple to elaborate, and drawing on a variety of ethnic cuisines, they all showcase the exceptional creativity and scope of these talented chefs.

AMANDA COHEN

Part of the gourmet New York food world for years, in 2008 Amanda opened her own restaurant in New York's East Village and called it Dirt Candy. Known for her ability to cook vegetables in unique and innovative ways, in 2010 Amanda was a contestant on *Iron Chef America*. For more information, visit dirtcandy.com.

MATTHEW KENNEY

Matthew is a chef, a restaurateur, and an author, and is known for his unique brand of organic and vegetarian cuisine. His company, Matthew Kenney Cuisine, is focused on the development of products, books, and businesses that reflect his passion for sustainable living.

He is the founder and operator of The 105degrees Academy, which is a state-licensed educational institution. Matthew created it to share and advance cutting-edge "living cuisine" in an inviting environment.

For more information about Matthew, his many books, the 105degrees Academy, or his work in general, you may visit 105degreesacademy.com.

JULIE MORRIS

Julie Morris is a Los Angeles–based food writer and natural food chef with a talent for creating delicious, health-boosting, plant-based, whole-food recipes. As a chef, she combines complementary ingredients to achieve a unique yet balanced flavor profile in a remarkable way. Julie specializes in the creation of recipes using superfoods. Although a formal definition has not been settled upon, superfoods are most commonly recognized as foods with a high nutrient density.

For more information about Julie, or to read her blog, watch her recipe preparation videos, or learn about her new book, *Superfood Cuisine*, you may visit juliemorris.net.

CHAD SARNO

Currently the R&D chef for Whole Foods Markets' "Health Starts Here" program, Chad has been bringing his approach to healthy cuisine to some of the world's premier organic vegan restaurants, spa resorts, film sets, and individuals for over a decade. I was first exposed to Chad's creations when he was executive chef at Saf, a unique upscale raw restaurant in London, England, back in 2008. I've been a fan ever since.

To learn more about Chad, his work, and his company, Vital Creations, you may visit his site rawchef.com.

TAL RONNEN

Chef Tal Ronnen is one of the most celebrated plant-based chefs working today. In the spring of 2008, he became known nationwide as the chef who prepared plant-based meals for Oprah Winfrey's 21-day vegan cleanse. Chef Ronnen also has the honor of being the first to serve a plant-based dinner at the U.S. Senate. Catering the 2010 Physicians Committee for Responsible Medicine (PCRM) gala in Los Angeles, Tal prepared a diverse menu, which was my first exposure to his recipe-creating prowess.

To view Tal's videos and to learn more about him and his book, *The Conscious Cook,* you may visit talronnen.com.

Recipes from My Favorite Restaurants

Throughout the recipe section you'll also find recipes from my favorite restaurants and cafés across North America. Ranging from elaborate five-star formal dining, to casual cafés, and even to basic takeout, these establishments are top-tier and each offers a unique culinary experience, all paralleling my nutritional philosophy.

As someone who crisscrosses North America several times each year, in addition to appreciating the Whole Foods Market and other plant-based, whole food–savvy grocery stores, I have a few favorite restaurants and cafés:

- **Beets Living Foods Café**—Austin, Texas
- **Blossoming Lotus**—Portland, Oregon
- **Candle 79**—New York City, New York
- **Cru**—Los Angeles, California
- **Crudessence**—Montreal, Quebec
- **Fresh at Home**—Toronto, Ontario
- **Gorilla Food**—Vancouver, British Columbia
- **The Green Door**—Ottawa, Ontario
- **Horizons**—Philadelphia, Pennsylvania
- **JivamukTea Café**—New York City, New York
- **Karyn's on Green**—Chicago, Illinois
- **Karyn's Fresh Corner Café**—Chicago, Illinois
- **Life Food Gourmet**—Miami, Florida
- **Live Organic Food Bar**—Toronto, Ontario
- **Millennium**—San Francisco, California
- **Pure Food & Wine**—New York, New York
- **Ravens' Restaurant**—Mendocino, California
- **Thrive Juice Bar**—Waterloo, Ontario
- **Veggie Grill**—Los Angeles, California

You can find more information about each establishment, along with its website URL, address, and phone number, starting on page 302.

1 HEALTH'S DEPENDENCE ON NUTRITION

Stress: just thinking about it can bring it on. When the term was first used in the 1930s, it meant biological trauma, that is, an incident causing physical harm. But in recent decades, we have come to more commonly speak about stress in psychological terms. Its context changed to include the daily events of modern life, not just physical strain. "Modern life stress," as it is sometimes termed, while often originating with worry, or simply a feeling of being overwhelmed, is still displayed through physical symptoms.

In North America, the number of reported incidences of stress-related illness is steadily escalating, so to say that stress has become an epidemic is putting it mildly. Stress has been shown to be the catalyst for numerous diseases.[1] Before disease itself is manifested, our bodies will display warning signals in the form of health problems. However, most of us ignore these signs. Or worse, we treat them as though they are the whole problem, overlooking where they come from.

Sleep deprivation, fatigue, mental fog, irritability, weight gain, and sugar, starch, and caffeine cravings are not in themselves problems but rather symptoms of a problem. They are, however, the red flags that alert us that our overall stress level is beyond a healthy range.

To use a driving analogy, if the oil light goes on, you may be tempted to simply put a piece of tape over it. If you give in to your urge, you will no longer be visually alerted to the problem. But of course, the problem hasn't gone away. The problem will worsen until the car's engine seizes. A lit oil light is the mechanical equivalent of sugar cravings: the first sign that a problem is materializing. And while eating refined sugar will provide relief from the symptom, it will be short-lived. And, of course, the cause will remain unchecked.

REDUCING NUTRITIONAL STRESS

So, what does stress have to do with nutrition? That's exactly what I wondered when I began preparing (I hoped) to embark on a career as a full-time athlete. My aspiration was to race Ironman triathlons professionally. And I was willing to do whatever it took to make it happen. One thing it took, as you might expect, was a lot of training.

Over the years I had trained diligently and my fitness improved. But the rate at which I was improving was beginning to slow. Of course, as a person becomes proficient at something—anything—the rate of improvement will decline. However, it got to where my rate of improvement wasn't just declining but slowing to a halt. I had hit a plateau.

For the extraordinary amount of time and energy I was spending on training, the return I was now receiving in terms of enhanced fitness was modest at best. I had to try something different. I had to find a way to break through and advance to the next level.

But if not more training, what was it going to take? After a lot of research, I came across truly useful material. As I delved deeper into my investigation, I discovered what I needed to do to break out of my modest-at-best-gains rut. I had to increase my rate of recovery, the speed at which cellular repair took place.

This became the focal point of my research and evolved into what would consume my next several years. I had become convinced that improved cellular regeneration after exercise would be my express ticket to success, and I began searching for ways to accelerate it. This was the key: I knew that quicker recovery would allow me to schedule workouts closer together and therefore to cram more training into a shorter amount of time.

And while I understood that food provides us with the fuel to move around, what I was just beginning to realize was that it also supplies us with the building blocks we use to reconstruct our bodies during the regeneration process. Cellular tissue is constantly dying and regenerating, but for those who break down muscle tissue at an extraordinary rate—athletes, for example, by way of exercise—nutritional building blocks enable the body to grow back stronger than it was pre-workout. Overcompensation by the body—its ability to grow stronger as a result of being broken down—is the training effect at work. But the body needs premium building blocks to regenerate in a timely and thorough manner. Fortunately for me, I had just realized—and still at a young age—that there was no such thing as overtraining, only under-recovering.

> The body needs premium building blocks to regenerate in a timely and thorough manner.

And, as I learned, nutrition—whether good or bad—plays a significant role in the regeneration process. Nutrition can speed it or slow it, depending on the quality of food. Adding to the physical strain of training, low-quality nutrition imposes stress of its own. And unlike the stress of training, from which the athlete receives a benefit (a greater level of fitness), the stress incurred from poor diet brings no gains. "Reducing stress by way of improved nutrition" was, in fact, the premise of my first book, *Thrive*.

When the body doesn't get the "biological building blocks"—the nutrients—it needs to keep pace with cellular regeneration, it experiences *nutritional stress*. And the body reacts to nutritional stress just as it does to mental or physical stress. The typical symptoms of stress begin to develop. It became apparent to me that taking in greater amounts of nutrients was a logical way to mitigate overall stress and therefore its symptoms.

My solution at first was simply to eat as much as I could. But, as I quickly learned the hard way, food is not necessarily synonymous with nutrition, at least not in the world we live in today.

What I had done was make sure I was fed, but unfortunately being fed is not the same as being nourished. There's a big difference. And my situation was in no way unique. In fact, I had just become average.

We North Americans are now an overfed yet undernourished society. Undernourishment is the new norm, no longer an exceptional state affecting only a small fraction of the population.

Here's how it works. Hunger is an essential, primal signal dating back to our earliest ancestors. Originating in our brain, the desire to eat is in fact a chemical signal triggered by the body's need for nutrients. To get fuel for our brain and muscles, as well as the building blocks for the ongoing repair of our cells, we need to eat. When we take in nutrient-rich food, such as fruit, our brain recognizes that we have responded to the chemical request it sent and turns off the signal, knowing that nourishment has been received. In the days when food was synonymous with nutrition, the more we ate, the better nourished we became. It really was that simple. That being the case, there was no desire to eat more than what we biologically required.

But times have changed. The highly refined foods that compose a large percentage of most North Americans' diet don't contain the nutritional components that would make them worthy of our consumption. These "foods" provide mass without sustenance. To make matters worse, they retain the calories. And calories without nutrients, also known as *low nutrient-dense food,* are the prime ingredients for a nutritional stress stew.

In *Thrive* I described my first exposure to significantly elevated stress, before I had discovered the major impact nutrition could have on regeneration. In one triathlon season in particular, the amount of training I was doing simply overwhelmed my system. It could not regenerate quickly enough to support the pace at which I was breaking it down. A high amount of physical stress, coupled with nutritional stress, elevated my level of cortisol (a stress hormone I'll tell you more about later), which then remained high for an extended period. After about four months, my stress problem had become chronic. I displayed all the telltale signs, but not understanding the relationship between stress and hormones, I ignored what I could and masked the rest: the general fatigue, difficulty sleeping, irritability, mental fog, and cravings for sugar and starchy food. While these symptoms of rampant stress were bothersome, they weren't nearly as debilitating for me as an athlete as those that were about to unfold. I actually began to gain weight. And it was *fat.* I was getting fatter, even though I was training full-time. The "experts" I consulted assured me the solution was simple: "If you're gaining fat, there can be only one reason—you're simply taking in more calories than what you're burning. Cut back on the amount you're eating and you'll lose weight."

This seemed odd to me. True, I was consuming a lot of food. But I had a hard time believing that it was in excess of what I was burning to fuel my significant volume of training. However, I was confused and out of ideas. So I tried the "experts'" suggestion. I cut back on the amount I ate.

What was to develop next I did not expect. Unbelievably, I began gaining weight even *more* quickly. Imagine: there I was, training 35 to 40 hours every single week, hardly eating, and *gaining* fat. How could that be?

> ✳ Second only to overconsumption, the greatest reason for obesity in North America is that we are simply inundated with more stress than our adrenal glands can deal with in a sustainable, healthy manner.

It wasn't until about a year and a half later that the answer was revealed. After speaking with an endocrinologist—a scientist with a deep understanding of the intricate relationship between stress and hormones—it became clear to me that I had placed too much strain on my adrenal glands, burned them out, and, as a result, was "hormonally injured." Elevated cortisol affects all other hormones, and as a result, balance—homeostasis—in the endocrine system falters. Additionally—and most significantly—when cortisol is elevated, it becomes nearly impossible to tone muscle or lose fat. In extreme cases, the body gains weight and loses muscle. And that's exactly what was happening in my situation.

As I learned the hard way, when I restricted the amount I ate, I gained fat rapidly because I wasn't getting adequate nutrition. My body desperately craved more nutrients, to help it cope with stress. Depriving my body of the nutrients it needed created greater nutritional stress and therefore more overall stress. Increased stress drove my cortisol levels higher, as my body sought to alleviate its stress through its own means. The higher my cortisol levels, the faster the symptoms of stress developed, such as fat gain.

My stress had come from the demands of training—physical stress. But excessive exercise is not the only cause of adrenal fatigue, and full-time athletes are not the only people at risk for elevated cortisol. The demands of modern life have the same cortisol-raising potential as physical stress. And as such, most North Americans have elevated cortisol levels—many with adrenal burnout—which prevent the body from toning muscle and burning fat effectively, despite regular exercise. Affecting more than 85 percent of North America's population, stress has reached never-before-seen levels. Second only to overconsumption (brought about by nutrient-absent food, as I explain on page 37), the greatest reason for obesity in North America is that we are simply inundated with more stress than our adrenal glands can deal with in a sustainable, healthy manner. But nutrient-dense whole foods can alleviate a considerable amount of that stress. And with lower stress come less severe and fewer symptoms.

The reality is that work, family, and the other stressors in our lives are sometimes not within our control. Fortunately, what we choose to eat is. Therefore, we can have a commanding influence on our overall stress levels. Once we have lowered our overall stress by eating well, we can more easily address some of the other daunting issues causing us traditional stress. But nutrition is a good place to start, and plant-based nutrient-dense whole foods are the base. The recipes in Chapter 6 encompass all the nutritional building blocks to ensure that nutritional stress is the least of your worries.

NUTRITION'S INFLUENCE ON SLEEP

We all know sleep is important and that without enough our mental and physical performance deteriorates. Brain function sharply declines, decision-making becomes labored, and reasoning escapes us. Our bodies don't repair the previous day's cellular wear and tear—the broken-down body tissue—in a timely fashion if we don't get enough rest, and stiffness and weakness are the result.

> Delta-phase sleep is possible only when one's cortisol level is low.

As reported by several studies, people who get at least eight hours of sleep a night are not as susceptible to contracting disease, have a greater ability to focus, and are less prone to developing depression than those who sleep less. It's such findings that prompt "experts" to suggest that most of us "should sleep more."[2] I, however, suggest it's not *more* sleep that most of us need but *better-quality* sleep. To be specific, most of us need more deep delta-phase sleep. This is the phase in which growth hormone is released, naturally triggering cellular repair and regeneration.[3] To sleep in the delta phase is to sleep efficiently, and if we have plenty of delta-phase sleep, we need less total sleep. Unfortunately, the vast majority of North Americans aren't able to slip into the delta phase. Their stress level, and therefore their cortisol, is simply too high to let them. Physiologically, it's impossible to enter the delta phase while cortisol is elevated. Realizing the full restorative properties of sleep requires lowering our cortisol to a level few North Americans can reach without first significantly altering their diet.

Delta-phase sleep is possible only when one's cortisol level is low.

Clearly this relationship is a vicious circle. Stress prevents quality sleep so that we then need more sleep to compensate for its poor quality. Or fatigue takes hold, which we remedy with stimulants in the form of caffeine or sugar. Yes, more sleep will indeed help people feel better rested and acquire the benefits listed above. However, lower cortisol will enable more *efficient* sleep, and therefore not as much will be required to facilitate quick regeneration and the benefits that come with it.

Speaking biologically, improving sleep efficiency will reduce the quantity requirement. That's good. Those extra waking hours give us more time to spend as we please—provided, of course, we're alert and functioning at a high level, both mentally and physically. In order to be high functioning, we need to be well rested. So, although sleep is a central component of health and wellness, it is not the duration that is of utmost importance, it's the quality.

As you've undoubtedly noticed, the line between being awake and being asleep has become blurred for many people. Once the fleeting stimulation of coffee and sugar wears off, these people spend their days in a state of mental haze. Even after eight hours of sleep, they wake up feeling both physically and mentally tired. And it shows. Have you ever had a conversation with someone and asked yourself, "Is this person awake?" The answer is probably "not completely." Because when this person was sleeping, he or she probably wasn't completely asleep either, at least not in the deep, refreshing delta phase. And because that person couldn't sleep deeply, because of high levels of overall stress, he or she also couldn't be fully focused, alert, and present when awake. Of course, it's in our best interest to sharply define that line. When we sleep, we want to be completely and deeply asleep so that when we're awake, we can function optimally.

Because of the undeniable restorative value of high-quality sleep, there's been a long-running debate as to what's more important for overall health: high-quality nutrition or high-quality sleep.

On the one hand, nutrition provides building material to replace aging cells with new, vibrant ones. A nutrient-dense diet also reduces nutritional stress. On the other hand, high-quality delta-phase sleep is when that repair actually takes place. And high-quality deep sleep can occur only when cortisol levels are low. Since nutrient-dense food reduces stress, a healthy diet improves cortisol levels and thus the quality of sleep. Better rested people do not crave sugary and starchy foods, since they simply do not require their stimulating energy. And in turn, high-quality sleep makes it easier to maintain a healthy diet.

So I think it's safe to say that neither high-quality sleep nor nutrient-dense food is *more* important to health but that they are complementary; the benefit of each is enhanced by the other. All the same, a person needs to have his or her nutrition needs met through quality food, or the delta-phase sleep can't be had at all.

High-quality sleep is imperative for high-quality living. And to achieve high-quality sleep we require high-quality, nutrient-dense food.

Deep delta-phase sleep is necessary for efficient cellular restoration. Nutrient-dense food is necessary for delta sleep.

Those who base their diet on low nutrient-dense foods have to eat more to become equally nourished, which means the consumption of more calories without an increase in nutrition. This pattern leads to chronic hunger and, most likely, weight gain.

NUTRIENT DENSITY: WHAT IT IS AND WHY IT MATTERS

Known as macronutrients, protein, carbohydrate, and fat together compose—in varying ratios—100 percent of the calorie content in all foods (sugar, fiber, and starch are types of carbohydrate). This being the case, eating anything edible is a guarantee that you'll obtain macronutrients.

Altering the ratio of macronutrients is a strategy used by athletes in pursuit of specific goals. For example, increasing the fat and protein ratios (eating more fat and protein) during endurance training will help improve fat metabolism and prevent muscle breakdown. More protein and starchy carbohydrates, such as sweet potatoes, will help to volumize and build muscles in strength athletes. A diet higher in sugar (in the form of fruit) will provide easily digestible sustenance to athletes in need of quick energy immediately prior to short intense workouts. In *Thrive*, I explain these athletic fueling strategies in detail.

However, the term "nutrient density" does not refer to macronutrients but to micronutrients. Unlike macronutrients, micronutrients contain *no* calories. There is also no guarantee that food will contain them. In fact, as I explain in detail in Chapter 3, since the quality of the soil in which the food is grown determines its micronutrient content—based on the soil mineral content—a large percentage of our modern food supply lacks micronutrients because of over-farming. That's a problem.

The World Health Organization agrees, referring to micronutrients as the "'magic wands' that enable the body to produce enzymes, hormones and other substances essential for proper growth and development."[4]

All vitamins, minerals, trace minerals, phytochemicals, antioxidants, and carotenoids are classified as micronutrients. Other than protein, carbohydrate, and fat, every nutritional component is that of a micronutrient. A complete list of known micronutrients (it's theorized there are many yet to be discovered), along with the role each plays, can be found in "Guide to Nutrients" on page 293. As you can see, the list is extensive. And since micronutrients are the backbone of nutrition itself, their

> A simple ratio, a food's nutrient density can be calculated by dividing the combined and averaged micronutrient content in any given food by the number of calories it contains.

dietary presence will dramatically reduce nutritional stress and therefore the symptoms that accompany it.

In fact, in 2005 the United States Department of Agriculture (USDA) published a report suggesting that we in North America consume too many calories and too few micronutrients, and that as a consequence our health is steadily declining.[5] Recognizing that consuming food no longer guarantees nutrient intake, in an uncharacteristically progressive move, the USDA came up with a simple yet effective way to help people view food in a different light. Nutrient content is what we ought to seek from food, not calories. In fact, the report urged, the more nutrients we can get from our food while taking in fewer calories in the process, the better. "Nutrient density" emerged as *the* food attribute to seek. A simple ratio, a food's nutrient density can be calculated by dividing the combined and averaged micronutrient content in any given food by the number of calories it contains. Since micronutrients are expressed in several different measurements (milligrams, micrograms, and international units), each was converted into a percentage of the USDA's recommended daily intake (RDI), to establish a benchmark and provide a starting point for the calculation. And while I don't necessarily agree with the percentages of RDI put forth by the USDA, their established values serve nicely as a means by which to institute a consistent benchmark.

In the years that followed, Dr. Joel Fuhrman, the author of an excellent book entitled *Eat to Live,* took the nutrient density ratio one step further and factored in antioxidants (which include phytonutrients, or phytochemicals, compounds found naturally in plants), for which there are currently no USDA recommended daily intakes. Yet their role in obtaining optimal health is well established as vital; as such, Dr. Fuhrman wisely includes them when calculating nutrient density values for various foods.[6]

Additionally, the USDA's evaluation system falls short in that phytonutrients have been shown to contain disease-fighting and anti-inflammation properties. Clearly, these nutritional compounds have value that should be factored into nutrient density scoring.

Interestingly, plants grown with herbicides and pesticides—rendering them non-organic—no longer need to develop compounds to defend themselves from weeds, insects, and other pests, because added chemicals now fill that role.[7] The disadvantage of this development—besides the synthetic chemical residue on our food—is that the self-protecting compounds plants would have naturally produced to make them undesirable to insects are in fact powerful phytonutrients.

Overall, because Dr. Fuhrman includes antioxidants in his nutrient-density calculation method, I believe it to be of greater value than the one originally put forth by the USDA. For this reason, when we assess nutrient density in Chapter 3, I have chosen to use his system.

However, by applying the Guiding Principles (beginning on page 21), we remove complicated calculations from the equation and simplify the pursuit of nutrient-dense foods. In addition, when food choices are plant-based whole foods, there is simply no need to count, or even observe, calories or grams of macronutrients. Basing the diet on plant-based whole foods will ensure everything falls into place. But before moving on to the Guiding Principles, let's look at a couple of areas where my whole-food Thrive diet, based on nutrient density, and a conventional diet, based on calorie counting, diverge significantly: fat and portion control.

High-Quality Raw Fat

Conventional diets say that fat is bad. And since fat contains more calories than carbohydrate or protein, it's true that even the healthiest fatty foods tend to be slightly less nutrient dense. However, the extra calories from high-quality fat can provide a benefit that offsets their slightly lower nutrient density.

Sources of fat that are unrefined, plant-based, and raw offer benefits in the form of omega-6 and omega-3 "essential" fatty acids (EFAs). These fatty acids are termed "essential" because the body needs them for peak health but can't manufacture them on its own—they must be obtained through food.

Those who take in adequate amounts of essential omega-3 and omega-6 fatty acids through their diet and who have them in correct balance have a lower risk of developing cardiovascular disease, diabetes, and arthritis.[8] The good news is that a diet comprised of plant-based whole foods delivers plenty of omega-6 and omega-3 as a matter of course. The ideal ratio of omega-6 to omega-3, namely, 2:1 to 4:1 (two to four times more omega-6 than omega-3) will automatically fall into place. Smoother, more supple skin and more efficient metabolism of fat are two immediate benefits that the correct balance of omega-3 and omega-6 EFAs in the diet bring.

Of course, an efficient fat metabolism directly translates into a leaner frame and—for the athlete—greater endurance during training sessions and races lasting two hours or more. Most raw nuts and seeds are an excellent source of high-quality fat. Although omega-3 is more difficult to come by than omega-6, excellent sources are flaxseeds, hemp seeds, chia, and, in particular, a seed called sacha inchi (what I classify as a "next-level food"). I'll be telling you more about these foods in Chapter 5, "Nutrient-Dense Whole Foods to Thrive," and of course the recipes in Chapter 6 offer several ways to make them part of your diet, too.

Nuts and seeds tend to score marginally lower on the nutrient density scale only because of their slightly greater fat content, not because of a lack of micronutrient levels. Interestingly, while hemp seeds and flaxseeds are full of micronutrients, their pressed oil is not. It's pure fat with very few micronutrients. Despite that, their oil is a worthy addition to your diet for its high levels of health-promoting omega-3 and omega-6 essential fatty acids. Coconut oil is another example that delivers more than you might expect. While it's not high in essential fatty acids, it is packed with medium chain triglycerides (MCT), a premium source of non-adrenal-stimulating fuel. I use coconut oil for its high-octane energy in several of my pre-workout, sport-specific recipes. (See Chapter 5 for more on coconut oil and MCTs.)

In short, cold-pressed, unrefined, plant-based seed and coconut oils are the exceptions to the nutrient-density rule.

As you'll notice, most of the salad dressing and sauce recipes in Chapter 6 are based on these oils.

Portion Control

Since I'm an advocate of nutrient-dense whole foods, I am not a supporter of portion control. The two simply can't coexist. If we eat nutrient-dense food, our chemical hunger signal will turn off naturally, as it did for our earliest ancestors. To forcefully deny ourselves continued eating when we desire to consume more is a reaction and a testament to our nutrient-lacking food. Forced portion control is nothing more than a symptom of a systemic problem that has been breed by our unhealthy farming system and our misguided focus on food volume production as opposed to food nutrient density (which I explain in detail, starting on page 16). By means of pesticides and genetic modification, an artificially created abundance of food volume leads to one

> When there's a lack of micronutrients in what we eat, our hunger signal remains active; overconsumption and weight gain are likely the result.

thing: a poverty of micronutrients. And, as we know, when there's a lack of micronutrients in what we eat, our hunger signal remains active; overconsumption and weight gain are likely the result.

I grew up in a wooded area in North Vancouver, and each spring I had a front-row seat to watch what happened when black bears stopped eating a natural, nutrient-rich diet and began literally eating garbage. Black bears wandering down from the forest in search of easily obtainable food would feed on garbage left on the curb for pickup. Food scraps were what they sought out in the suburban curbside disposal bins. High in calories, easy to obtain, and addictive, the processed human food would hook the bears. And in becoming hooked, the bears, just like humans, became lethargic and began packing on the pounds. By summer, they were undeniably tired and fat.

The only difference between these suburban garbage eaters and their counterparts in the forest was what they were eating. Instead of their natural diet—nutrient-rich roots, buds, berries, dandelions, and fruit—the suburban visitors were eating one that mirrored ours, high in calories, low in nutrients. And bears aren't the only wild animals to undergo this transformation when they begin eating our calorie-laden, nutrient-absent food. Raccoons, coyotes, and mountain lions—none are immune to the effects of low-quality food. And before long, as with humans on this diet, they become portly and lethargic.

Our preoccupation with producing a greater volume of food, rather than more nutritious food (I discuss the implications of this blinkered view of food production in detail in Chapter 2), is ultimately the culprit. And portion control can't fix the problem of undernourishment.

GUIDING PRINCIPLES

The Guiding Principles I set out below are five fundamental nutritional ideas that build on the premise of eating nutrient-dense, plant-based whole foods. These principles go hand in hand with my nutritional philosophy and are here to guide you when you're faced with making choices about what to eat. Of course, all the recipes in this book adhere to these principles.

My Five Thrive Guiding Principles

1. Eliminate biological debt: acquire energy through nourishment not stimulation.
2. Go for high-net-gain foods: make a small investment for a big return.
3. Aim for a high percentage of raw and low-temperature-cooked foods.
4. Choose alkaline-forming foods.
5. Avoid common allergens.

1. ELIMINATE BIOLOGICAL DEBT: ACQUIRE ENERGY THROUGH NOURISHMENT NOT STIMULATION

Biological debt is the term I use to describe the unfortunate, energy-depleted state that North Americans frequently find themselves in. Often brought about by eating refined sugar or drinking coffee to gain short-term energy, biological debt is the ensuing energy "crash."

There are two types of energy: one obtained from stimulation, the other from nourishment. The difference between the two is clear-cut. Stimulation is short-term energy and simply treats the symptom of fatigue. Being well nourished, in contrast, eliminates the need for stimulation, because a steady supply of energy is available to those whose nutritional needs have been met. In effect, sound nutrition is a preemptive strike against fatigue and the ensuing desire for stimulants. With nutrient-dense whole food as the foundation of your diet, there's no need to ever get into biological debt.

Generally speaking, the more a food is *fractionalized* (the term used to describe a once-whole food that has had nutritional components removed), the more stimulating its effect on the nervous system. And of course there's also caffeine to consider, North Americans' second-favorite drug (next to refined sugar). By way of stimulation, fractionalized foods and caffeinated beverages boost energy nearly immediately. But almost as quickly, within only a few hours, that energy will be gone. It is a short-term, unsustainable solution to the *symptom* of our energy debt. Adrenal gland stimulation *always* carries a cost. Obtaining energy by way of stimulation is like shopping with a credit card. You get something you desire now but that doesn't mean you won't have to pay eventually. The "bill" will come. And with that bill comes incurred biological interest: fatigue. Again.

We tend to rely upon additional stimulation to deal with this second wave of weariness, which in turn simply delays the moment when we pay off our tab. But the longer we put off payment, the greater the debt we accumulate. To continue our debt/credit analogy, to simply continue to summon energy by way of stimulation is like paying off one credit card with another. All the while, the interest is mounting.

Stimulation is a bad substitute for nourishment for another reason. It makes demands on the adrenal glands, prompting the production of the stress hormone cortisol. Elevated cortisol is linked to inflammation,[9] which is a concern for the athlete (and for anyone who appreciates fluid movement). Higher levels of cortisol also weaken cellular tissue, lower immune response, increase the risk of disease, cause body tissue degeneration, reduce sleep quality, and are a catalyst for the accumulation of body fat.[10] As if that weren't enough, chronic elevated levels of cortisol *reduce* the effectiveness of exercise, activity that normally helps to keep cortisol in check. Too-high cortisol levels can actually break down muscle tissue, as well as prevent the action of other hormones that build muscle. As a result, muscles not only become more difficult to tone but strength is likely to decline rather than increase.

Not surprisingly, if we keep on overstimulating our overstressed body, without addressing the real problem behind our fatigue, things only get worse. The severity of the symptoms of stress increase so that our health declines little by little. We put ourselves at greater risk for serious disease.

Often the first symptom of adrenal fatigue is increased appetite, followed by cravings, commonly for starchy, refined foods; difficulty sleeping; irritability; mental fog; lack of motivation; body fat gain; lean muscle loss; visible signs of premature aging; and sickness.[11] If this cycle of chronically elevated cortisol levels is allowed to continue, tissue degeneration, depression, chronic fatigue syndrome, and even diseases such as cancer can develop.

> Energy derived from good nutrition—cost-free energy—does not take a toll on the adrenal glands and so doesn't need to be "stoked" with stimulating substances.

In contrast, when we use nutrient-dense whole food as our source of energy, rather than fleeting pick-me-ups, our adrenals will not be stimulated, and, simultaneously, our sustainable energy level will rise because of the acquired nutrients. Energy derived from good nutrition—cost-free energy—does not take a toll on the adrenal glands and so doesn't need to be "stoked" with stimulating substances. In fact, one characteristic of wellness is a ready supply of *natural* energy that doesn't rely on adrenal stimulation. People who are truly well have boundless energy with no need for stimulants, such as caffeine or refined sugar.

A cornerstone of my dietary philosophy is to break dependency on adrenal stimulation. As you might expect, we accomplish this by way of nutrient-dense whole foods. And not just by supplementing our diet with them but by *basing* our diet on them. This diet, along with proper rest through efficient sleep (efficient because of our reduced stress, thanks to nutrient-dense food), will address the *cause* of the problem, not just the *symptoms* of nutritional shortfalls.

2. GO FOR HIGH-NET-GAIN FOODS: MAKE A SMALL INVESTMENT FOR A BIG RETURN

High-net-gain foods deliver us energy by way of conservation as opposed to consumption. Here's what I mean by that: the digestive and assimilation process is in fact an energy-intensive one. At the onset of eating, we begin spending digestive resources in an effort to convert energy stored within food—also known as calories—into usable sustenance to fulfill our biological requirements. And, as we know, whenever energy is transferred from one form to another, there's an inherent loss. However, the amount of energy lost in this process varies greatly and depends on the foods eaten.

Highly processed, refined, denatured "food" requires that significantly more digestive energy be spent to break it down in the process of transferring its caloric energy to us:

$$\text{net energy gain} = \text{energy remaining}$$
$$\text{once digestive energy has been spent.}$$

While it's true that a calorie is a measure of food energy, simply eating more calories will not necessarily ensure more energy for the consumer. If there were such a calorie guarantee, people who subsisted on fast food and other such calorie-laden fare would have abundant energy. And of course they don't. This is a testament to the inordinate amount of digestive energy required to convert such "food" into usable fuel.

(By the way, it's no coincidence that the cultures that have their largest, heaviest meals for lunch are the same ones who have afternoon siestas. Digestion is tiring.)

In contrast, natural, unrefined whole food digests with a considerably lower energy requirement. Therefore, we can gain more usable energy from simply eating foods that are in a more natural whole state, even if they have fewer calories.

When I grasped this concept, I began viewing food consumption as though it were an investment of sorts. My goal became to spend, or invest, as little digestive energy as possible to acquire the greatest amount of micronutrients and maximize the return on my investment.

For that reason, I refer to foods that require little digestive energy but yield a healthy dose of micronutrients as high-net-gain foods:

high net gain = little digestive energy spent,
substantial level of micronutrients gained.

With this principle in mind, I shifted my prime carbohydrate sources from processed and refined carbs, such as pasta and bread, to fruit. Fruit is packed with carbohydrate in the form of easily assimilated sugar, considerably easier to digest than refined grain flour. And fruit returns higher micronutrient levels than these processed, refined carb sources.

3. AIM FOR A HIGH PERCENTAGE OF RAW AND LOW-TEMPERATURE-COOKED FOODS

Foods that have not been heated above 118 degrees Fahrenheit are termed raw. There are several advantages to eating a large quantity of raw food in place of its cooked counterpart. Ease of digestion and assimilation, which directly translates into additional energy by means of an increase in net gain, is the most significant. Enzymes that contribute to overall health and aid digestion are not present in cooked food; heating above

118 degrees Fahrenheit destroys them. Before the body can turn cooked food into usable fuel, it must produce enzymes to aid in the digestion process. A healthy person can create these enzymes, but it costs energy, which creates a nominal amount of stress. As well, as we get older, our enzyme production naturally slows down; if we are not getting enough enzyme-rich foods in our regular diet, our enzyme-production system will have to work even harder. Overtaxing the system can weaken it further and lead to major digestive problems. Including enzyme-rich foods in our diet on a regular basis will help safeguard our bodies' ability to manufacture enzymes. Interestingly, a person who cannot produce digestive enzymes and does not obtain them through food can acquire the same diseases as someone suffering from malnutrition.[12]

> Food cooked at a high temperature can cause inflammation.

At only slightly above 118 degrees Fahrenheit, enzyme quality in food will sharply drop off. The next significant quality decline comes when food reaches a temperature of about 300 degrees Fahrenheit. This is the point at which essential fatty acids convert into trans fats. Additionally, food cooked at a high temperature can cause inflammation. When sugar is heated to a high temperature with fat, it can create end products known as AGEs (short for *advanced glycation end products*), which the body perceives as invaders. The immune cells try to break down these end products by secreting large amounts of inflammatory agents. If the cycle continues, it can result in problems commonly associated with old age: less elastic skin, arthritis, weakened memory, joint pain, and even heart disease.

Most of the base ingredients (the most common being corn, soy, or wheat flour) in refined foods on the typical grocery store shelf have been heated to well above 300 degrees. Because of this, the fat within those flours has become denatured and therefore is not only unusable by the body but perceived by the immune system as a threat, which weakens the body's reserves and causes a rise in cortisol.

As you will notice, many of the Thrive recipes in Chapter 6 are raw (look for the raw icon: 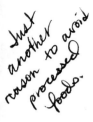). About 80 percent of my own diet is raw, and I find that percentage works well.

Just another reason to avoid processed foods.

4. CHOOSE ALKALINE-FORMING FOODS

The measure of acidity or alkalinity is called pH, and maintaining a balanced pH within the body is an important part of achieving and sustaining peak health. If our pH drops, our body becomes too acidic, adversely affecting health at the cellular level. People with low pH are prone to many ailments and to fatigue.

The body can become more acidic through diet and, to a lesser extent, stress. Since our bodies are equipped with buffering capabilities, our blood pH will vary to only a small degree, regardless of poor diet and other types of stress. But the other systems recruited to facilitate this buffering use energy and can become strained. Over time, the result of this buffering is significant stress on the system, which causes immune function to falter, effectively opening the door to a host of diseases.

> ✳ Minerals are exceptionally alkaline-forming, so foods with a greater concentration of micronutrients—greater nutrient density—will inherently have a greater alkaline-forming effect.

Low body pH can lead to the development of kidney stones, loss of bone mass, and the reduction of growth hormone, which results in loss of lean muscle mass and increase in body fat production. And since a decline in growth hormone production directly results in lean muscle tissue loss and body fat gain, the overconsumption of acid-forming foods plays a significant role in North America's largest health crisis. However, food is not the only thing we put in our bodies that is acid-forming. Most prescription drugs, artificial sweeteners, and synthetic vitamin and mineral supplements are extremely acid-forming.

Low body pH is also responsible for an increase in the fabrication of cell-damaging free radicals and a loss in cellular energy production. Free radicals alter cell membranes and can adversely affect our DNA.

So what can we do to prevent all this? The answer is to consume more alkaline-forming foods and fewer acid-forming ones.

Minerals are exceptionally alkaline-forming, so foods with a greater concentration of micronutrients—greater nutrient density—will inherently have a greater alkaline-forming effect.

Another factor that significantly raises the pH of food and, in turn, the body, is chlorophyll content.

Responsible for giving plants their green pigment, chlorophyll is often referred to as the blood of plants. The botanical equivalent to hemoglobin in human blood, chlorophyll synthesizes energy. Chlorophyll converts the sun's energy that has been absorbed by the plant into carbohydrate. Known as photosynthesis, this process is responsible for life on Earth. Since animals and humans eat plants, we too get our energy from the sun, plants being the conduit. Chlorophyll is prized for its ability to cleanse our blood by helping remove toxins deposited from dietary and environmental sources. Chlorophyll is also linked to the body's production of red blood cells, making daily consumption of chlorophyll-rich foods important for ensuring the body's constant cell regeneration and for improving oxygen transport in the body and, therefore, energy levels. By optimizing the body's regeneration of blood cells, chlorophyll also contributes to peak athletic performance.

5. AVOID COMMON ALLERGENS

Causing, at the very least, symptoms such as mild nasal congestion, headache, and mental fog, sensitivities to certain foods are exceptionally common. Wheat, gluten (in wheat), corn, soy, and dairy are the most common of these allergens.

A sensitivity is an unpleasant reaction caused by eating food for which the body lacks the specific enzymes or chemicals to digest it properly. Unlike an allergic reaction, a sensitivity does not affect the immune system. Food allergies often become evident immediately upon consuming the food: there's no mistaking an allergic reaction, which comes on quickly and often violently, ranging all the way from abdominal cramps and vomiting or a tingling in the mouth, to life-threatening anaphylactic shock, with swelling of the tongue and throat and difficulty breathing. As serious as an allergic reaction may be, once the allergen is identified, the solution is straightforward: don't eat the food again! The symptoms of a specific food sensitivity, however, may not become evident for a few days or even a week after consumption, making its source difficult to trace. Food sensitivities, therefore, can be extremely difficult to immediately identify and eliminate, and in these cases, the strategy of eliminating common allergens from the diet is useful.

For several years, I had what I thought to be a bad case of hay fever. Each spring I would display the classic symptoms of pollen-caused allergies: dry eyes, sinus congestion, and mild flu-like symptoms. Thinking there was little I could do short of taking antihistamine drugs, which I wanted to avoid, I just put up with it. Since these symptoms flared up at the same time each year, it seemed obvious they must be related to environmental changes because of the onset of spring and the bursts of pollen in the air. Or so I thought.

When I began learning about sensitivities to food, I reanalyzed my diet. What I found intrigued me. Each year, as the winter turned to spring, I'd ramp up my cycling mileage in preparation for the coming triathlon season. And as the cycling ramped up, so did my consumption of the sports drink I sipped while logging the miles. My sports drink's base ingredient was maltrodextrin, which is an inexpensive form of carbohydrate, derived from corn. I got tested for food sensitivity, and sure enough, corn registered as one. Fresh, non-genetically modified corn on the cob didn't bother me, but corn in the highly processed state of maltrodextrin triggered an adverse reaction in my body.

From that point on, I began making my own sports drinks. You can find recipes for the original one I came up with, as well as some newer varieties, in the "Drinks" section in Chapter 6.

This discovery made me realize that many people have a food sensitivity—or several sensitivities—but they just don't know it. "Not feeling quite up to par" is their common description of their life in general. They rule out diet as the culprit since it's been a constant in their life—virtually unchanged—for years. Some people, as I did, blame environmental factors, such as dust or pollen. These annoying, low-grade symptoms, or sometimes a more general state of malaise, can go on or regularly recur for years; because the symptoms make just certain activities a bit more difficult without actually preventing them, the sufferer takes no action. But it is precisely the unchanging diet that is behind the symptoms.

If you suspect you may have a food sensitivity, try eliminating the common allergens—processed corn, wheat/gluten, dairy products, and soy—from your diet. Test by removing one food at a time for a period of 10 days so that you can isolate your reactions. If your symptoms subside when you are off the food, then you will know that it causes you problems and you'd be better off removing it from your diet. If you don't notice a change when you go off a food, then you can carry on eating it. It's that simple.

By the way, it's unlikely you'll find any processed, refined food at the supermarket that doesn't contain at least one of these common allergens. Corn and soy are particularly ubiquitous. They're cheap, shelf-stable, and take on other flavors well, so, in the eyes of the manufacturer, they're the perfect set of ingredients to increase the volume of processed foods, essentially being used as "filler," adding little to no nutritional value.

As described in this chapter, the implications of nutritional stress that results from a diet comprised of nutrient-absent foods can have a profound effect on us as individuals. In the next chapter, we'll look at the implications beyond the personal—to the effects on our environment of our food choices.

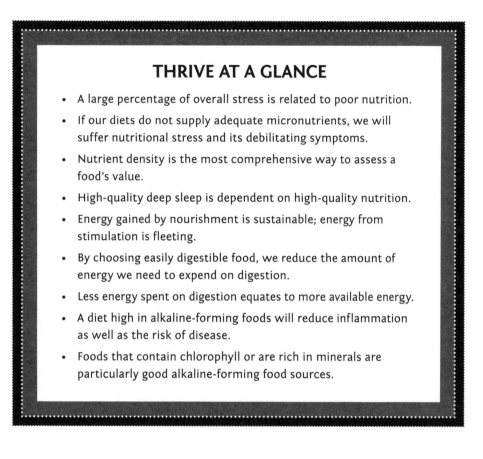

THRIVE AT A GLANCE

- A large percentage of overall stress is related to poor nutrition.
- If our diets do not supply adequate micronutrients, we will suffer nutritional stress and its debilitating symptoms.
- Nutrient density is the most comprehensive way to assess a food's value.
- High-quality deep sleep is dependent on high-quality nutrition.
- Energy gained by nourishment is sustainable; energy from stimulation is fleeting.
- By choosing easily digestible food, we reduce the amount of energy we need to expend on digestion.
- Less energy spent on digestion equates to more available energy.
- A diet high in alkaline-forming foods will reduce inflammation as well as the risk of disease.
- Foods that contain chlorophyll or are rich in minerals are particularly good alkaline-forming food sources.

EATING RESOURCES: The Environmental Toll of Food Production

Producing the vast amount of food required to support our population places a significant draw on our ecosystem, but it's a necessary exchange. Nonetheless, the divide between the resource requirements of plant-based food production and those of animal-based food production is impressive, greater than I ever could have imagined.

In the pages that follow, I explore the use of natural resources in relation to food production. The three natural resources required to produce food are arable land, water, and fuel (most of it fossil fuel). I also factor in the carbon dioxide, or CO_2, emissions that are released into the atmosphere through the burning of fossil fuel during the food production process. In addition, I consider other emission sources such as methane and nitrous oxide.

ARABLE LAND

Arable land refers to land that can be used for growing crops. It is undoubtedly one of our most precious natural resources and without it we couldn't produce even close to enough food to meet the demands of our rapidly growing population. While the land—the geographical space that croplands occupy—itself is vital, of equal importance is the quality of soil covering it.

Healthy topsoil is in fact a complex blend of elements that are vital to the growing process of nutritious food. Composed of a mixture of organic material, such as decaying plant matter, fungi, bacteria, and microorganisms, soil is much more than simply dirt. Just one acre can be home to 900 pounds of earthworms, 2400 pounds of fungi, 1500 pounds of bacteria, 133 pounds of protozoa, and 890 pounds of arthropods and algae.[1]

Topsoil also comprises a vast quantity of minerals that are the necessary catalysts for plants to produce vitamins, enzymes, antioxidants, a plethora of phytonutrients, and amino acids

> Plants are the medium. They draw minerals from the soil, passing them on to us in a form we can assimilate.

(protein), and that give them the ability to formulate hormones. Without minerals, none of these vital nutritional components can be constructed.

And since we can't digest soil, plants come to our aid; they draw minerals into their stalks, leaves, and seeds, and then act as the delivery system through which the nutrition originating in the soil (the minerals) is passed on to us, through the food we eat.

Plants are the medium. They draw minerals from the soil, passing them on to us in a form we can assimilate.

Minerals are not only vital for good health but are in fact the base on which health is built. Low mineral intake is now accepted as a substantial increased risk factor for myriad conditions, including osteoporosis, type 2 diabetes, depression, and obesity. Mineral deficiencies have been shown to play a role in cardiovascular disease (CVD), which kills 910,000 people in the United States annually.[2] That equates to an American death every 35 seconds. And while nutrient-absent food isn't the only contributing factor, it's among the most significant. According to the World Health Organization, a major reason for the widespread incidence of CVD is that "people are consuming a more energy-dense, nutrient-poor diet and are less physically active."[3] So basically people are eating more calories than they need while getting too few micronutrients—the textbook definition of a low nutrient-dense diet. In fact, two-time Nobel prize–winning chemist Dr. Linus Pauling stated that "you can trace every sickness, every disease and every ailment to a mineral deficiency."[4] As mentioned earlier, nutritional stress is primarily a result of a lack of micronutrients, such as minerals and phytonutrients, in our food, and they cannot be present in the food if minerals are lacking in the soil. And as we know, stress is the root cause of most diseases. And the lack of micronutrients in food is the root cause of nutritional stress. So good health actually begins in the soil.

Today, the mineral content in our soil is drastically lower than it was even just a few decades ago, contributing to the strange paradox of a population overfed yet undernourished, an increasing and widespread health issue. According to the findings at the United Nations Conference on Environment and Development (UNCED), also known as the Earth Summit, held in 1992, North America "leads" the continents of the world in soil mineral depletion, having lost 85 percent of the mineral content in its soil over the past century (in comparison, South America's and Asia's minerals are 76 percent of what they were 100 years ago; Africa's, 74 percent; Europe, 72 percent; and Australia, 55 percent).[5] Sodium, calcium, potassium, magnesium, phosphorus, copper, zinc, and iron—all of them began their taper about 100 years ago, as population growth began to strain the land and its ability to produce an adequate supply of food.

For reasons such as population growth, the demand we place on our dwindling supply of arable land continues to increase. As the population increases, not only are there more mouths to feed, but housing more people also leads to suburban sprawl, which paves over arable land. So, as our demand for food continued to grow, the geographic space in which to grow it continued to shrink.

Conventional farming has reacted to this dilemma with a simple objective: to grow as much food as possible on as little land as possible. Mass and volume of production became paramount, but unfortunately the quality of the food grown was neglected in the process.

Since traditionally food has been understood to be synonymous with nutrition, the thinking traditionally has been that the more food we eat, the better nourished we'll be. But, not so, as I explained in Chapter 1; I learned this the hard way when I tried to better nourish myself in hopes of propelling my athletic performance. I ate more food to try to correct my lack of nourishment, which led to being overfed yet undernourished, a condition that unfortunately affects a significant percentage of the population. As I know now, I should have eaten not simply more food but more nutrient-dense food. The disconnect I and so many others have experienced is that though food once equalled nutrition, it's not necessarily so today. Not taking mineral content into account, conventional farming aims simply to produce more food on less land. Volume, mass, and calories are all that's considered when evaluating crop yield.

Because of heavy demands on the North American food system, genetic modification and widespread pesticide use have become the rule, not the exception. Despite the increasing awareness and popularity of organic food, its production worldwide pales in comparison to that of conventionally farmed and genetically modified organism (GMO) crops. According to Organic-World.net, only 0.8% percent of the world's total crops are grown without genetic modification and organically.[6] Clearly, a minuscule amount. Specifically looking to North America, Organic-World.net states that as of 2008 only 0.93 percent of Canadian crops were grown organically, only slightly better than the world average, while the United States' organic food crops registered at a dismal 0.6 percent. While genetic modification and chemical pest deterrents allow for a greater volume of food to be produced on less land, they may prove to cause serious health problems in years to come. And the decline of nutrient density is likely just one of the negative effects of producing our food this way. The possible complications of long-term GMO crops in our food supply are as yet unknown, and the effects on our health of chemical residue from pesticides are still to be determined.

Since there is a finite amount of each mineral in a given plot of land, the plants grown are limited by what is present in the soil. More plants doesn't mean more nutrition. The more food that's grown on a given plot of land, the less total amount of minerals each plant will contain, rendering each plant less nutrient dense. Clearly that's a problem.

Another factor is the type of crop. Each species of plant has a set limit as to how much of a given mineral it can draw into its cellulose. Here's how it works: when we eat food grown in over-farmed, mineral-depleted soil, to obtain the same amount of health-essential minerals, we need to consume more food. This of course equates to a greater intake of calories. In addition, the chemical hunger signal that I mentioned in Chapter 1 will remain active until it's satisfied that we've got the minerals—and the vitamins and the phytochemicals that the plant can produce only once it has drawn an adequate supply of the minerals from the soil—that we need to be healthy.

And if our body is not satisfied—and it won't be if the minerals aren't in the soil—it will urge us to eat more the only way it knows how: by making us hungry. So hunger doesn't necessarily mean we haven't eaten enough food. <u>More often than not, today hunger means we haven't eaten enough *nutrient-rich* food.</u>

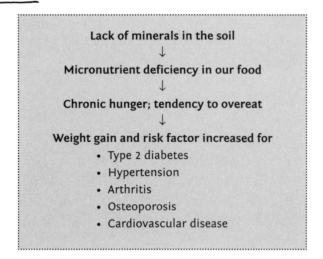

Lack of minerals in the soil
↓
Micronutrient deficiency in our food
↓
Chronic hunger; tendency to overeat
↓
Weight gain and risk factor increased for
- Type 2 diabetes
- Hypertension
- Arthritis
- Osteoporosis
- Cardiovascular disease

Since the consumption of more calories with fewer minerals leads to a chronically active hunger signal, the tendency to overeat, followed closely by weight gain, will be the result. Being overweight will increase the risk factor for a wide range of diseases: type 2 diabetes, hypertension, arthritis, osteoporosis, and cardiovascular disease. <u>So, simply producing a greater volume of food should not be our goal, but rather producing food that is of the highest nutrient density, which is governed, in large part, by soil quality.</u>

Why I want my own garden…

Clearly the consumption of more calories and fewer nutrients equates to a diet of lower nutrient density, which can lead to health concerns and disease. And in fact, it's what the Standard American Diet is built on: lots of calories but very few micronutrients, such as minerals.

Crop "yield" needs to be redefined and assessed as "nutrition contained within the food" as opposed to the total weight, volume, or caloric value of the food harvested.

Brian Halweil, a senior fellow at the Worldwatch Institute covering issues of food and agriculture, and the co-director of Nourishing the Planet, lays out the argument in a 2007 report titled *Still No Free Lunch: Nutrient Levels in U.S. Food Supply Eroded by Pursuit of High Yields*. Halweil describes the shortcomings of striving simply to obtain crop volume, mass, and calories from food. Instead, Halweil suggests, food producers ought to focus on the nutrient value of the food. Halweil eloquently concludes the report by saying:

> Yield increases per acre have come predominantly from two sources—growing more plants on a given acre, and harvesting more food or animal feed per plant in a given field. In some crops like corn, most of the yield increase has come from denser plantings, while in other crops, the dominant route to higher yields has been harvesting more food per plant, tree, or vine.
>
> But American agriculture's single-minded focus on increasing yields over the last half-century created a blind spot where incremental erosion in the nutritional quality of our food has occurred. This erosion, modest in some crops but significant in others for some nutrients, has gone largely unnoticed by scientists, farmers, government and consumers.[7]

Crop "yield" needs to be redefined and assessed as "nutrition contained within the food" as opposed to the total weight, volume, or caloric value of the food harvested.

Once I'd become familiar with the workings of this problem, the value of arable land was firmly impressed on me. I've never looked at rolling pastureland the same way since. What I learned next was hard to comprehend.

In 2008 I participated in the Students for Sustainability National Campus Tour, which was a joint initiative of the Canadian Federation of Students, the Sierra Youth Coalition, and the David Suzuki Foundation. We visited 22 campuses across Canada in 30 days, talking about the urgent need to create sustainable communities and campuses. While doing research for the speech I was preparing to deliver on the tour, I came across an extremely fascinating—and equally horrifying—piece of information. As unbelievable as it may seem, multiple reputable

> Livestock production uses a *staggering* 70 percent of all arable land and 30 percent of the land surface of the planet.

sources, such as the United Nations and the Worldwatch Institute, corroborated that 70 percent of the food grown on—and drawing minerals from—our precious arable land was not in fact for us to eat but would serve instead as animal food, specifically, livestock feed.[8]

Animals being raised to be eaten—and animals being raised so that their by-products can be eaten, such as cows for milk and chickens for eggs—are collectively termed livestock. According to the United Nations, the raising of livestock is by far the single greatest anthropogenic use of land. Twenty-six percent of the ice-free surface of Earth is used as grazing land. Additionally, 33 percent of total arable land is used to grow food—primarily corn, soy, and wheat—to feed to animals. Factoring in grazing land and feedcrop requirements, livestock production uses a *staggering* 70 percent of all arable land and 30 percent of the land surface of the planet.[9]

While soil mineral depletion began approximately 100 years ago, the sharpest decline started about 30 years later, beginning in the 1940s. Not so coincidentally, this is when large-scale animal agriculture began commandeering the vast majority of our land.

Also, since 1940, cardiovascular disease has been on the rise.[10] And interestingly, its escalation has been in concert with widespread animal agriculture and the corresponding decline of mineral-rich soil. Coincidence?

Unfortunately, even those who don't eat meat are impacted by inefficient farming because of loss of nutrient-rich soil, since it affects the whole food supply.

Note that the lack of mineral content in animal feed is not a concern—in fact, it's desirable. As with humans, when animals eat nutrient-absent refined starch-based calories, they gain weight. The whole point of feeding animals this grain-based diet is to quickly increase their mass. And that it does. Of course, as I've mentioned, if there are no nutrients in the soil, then there are none in the animal, or in the person who eats it.

Raising animals for food is clearly an exceptional draw on arable land. But, to make matters worse, it's also an incredibly inefficient way of utilizing the dwindling supply that remains. For example, for every 16 pounds of plant matter (primarily composed of corn, wheat, and soy, most of which is genetically modified) fed to a cow, one pound of meat is returned.[11] Where do the other 15 pounds go? While a fraction is burned to fuel the cow's movement and some is lost into the atmosphere in the form of heat, the vast

Sick money-hungry humans

majority ends up as manure. So, we are literally turning one of our most valuable natural resources into manure.

Currently, the livestock population in the United States consumes more than seven times as much grain as the human population eats.[12]

According to the U.S. Department of Agriculture, the amount of grain fed to U.S. livestock would be able to feed about 800 million people (2.7 times the entire U.S. population) who followed a plant-based diet.[13]

A factory-farmed cow needs to consume 16 pounds of cattle feed (wheat, corn, soy) to yield 1 pound of meat for human consumption.

Great Thought!

And that estimate's based on people simply eating the crops grown for livestock. Now, if instead of growing GMO corn, soy, and wheat—destined to be fed to animals—we were instead to sow the fields with non-GMO, organic, nutrient-rich crops, such as hemp, flax, yellow peas, and kale, we would not only be able to feed more than double the U.S. population with ease but, most importantly, we'd be feeding them with nutrient-dense whole food. Far fewer people would be overfed yet undernourished, and disease would significantly decline.

Factory-farmed animals are fed wheat, corn, and soy, which are primarily carbohydrate based. Yet because of the sheer volume these animals are fed, they ingest six times as much protein as they yield in return.[14] And it takes 20 times as much land to grow beef for protein as it does to grow plants for protein.

What about grass-fed beef? If all who ate factory-farmed beef were to switch to grass-fed, there simply would not be enough meat to go around. Factory farming was created for a reason: to produce more food on less land. And it works. However, as already pointed out, it does so by yielding volume, mass, and calories rather than the true components of nutrition.

If beef eaters in the United Sates were to switch to exclusively grass-fed beef, one small steak about once every three weeks is all that would be available. There simply wouldn't be enough to meet demand. And if more grazing land were to be created, of course deforestation would be the result.

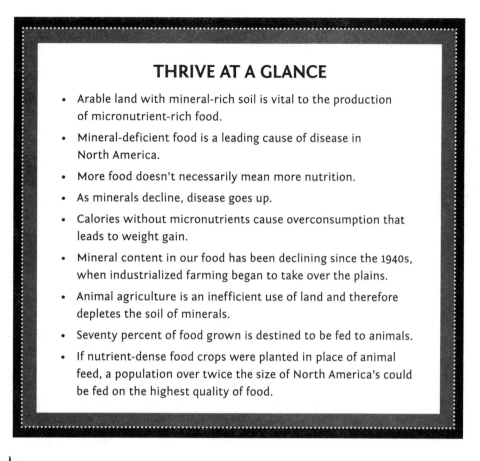

THRIVE AT A GLANCE

- Arable land with mineral-rich soil is vital to the production of micronutrient-rich food.
- Mineral-deficient food is a leading cause of disease in North America.
- More food doesn't necessarily mean more nutrition.
- As minerals decline, disease goes up.
- Calories without micronutrients cause overconsumption that leads to weight gain.
- Mineral content in our food has been declining since the 1940s, when industrialized farming began to take over the plains.
- Animal agriculture is an inefficient use of land and therefore depletes the soil of minerals.
- Seventy percent of food grown is destined to be fed to animals.
- If nutrient-dense food crops were planted in place of animal feed, a population over twice the size of North America's could be fed on the highest quality of food.

And as we know, it makes sense to "be the change we want to see in the world." So what if North Americans made the switch to eat grass-fed beef instead of factory-farmed meat? Would the result be a change we want to see? While one problem would be solved, another problem would arise—lack of grazing land. Clearly, swapping one problem for another will not give us a sustainable solution. We need to make the change—to be the change—that is a true, lasting solution.

FRESH WATER

Having grown up in North Vancouver and having rain fall from the sky for most of the year, learning to appreciate the value of water wasn't always easy. But in October 2008, while on the Students for Sustainability National Campus Tour, I met Maude Barlow. She is an author, an activist, and a world authority on water, and served as senior advisor to the United Nations. Understandably, I was honored to speak before her talk at Dalhousie University in Halifax, Nova Scotia.

After my speech, I sat back, watched, and listened. Barlow clearly articulated facts about water that I had never even considered. And as I began to see how the rest of the world lived—without water for proper sanitation or even adequate water to drink—I developed a newfound appreciation for it.

> Usable non-polluted fresh water is less than 1 percent of the Earth's total. And 70 percent of that 1 percent is primarily used for agriculture animal feed.

Referring to the much greater public concern about our looming energy crisis, Barlow stated that "no one ever died from a lack of energy."

That prompted me to delve deeper to find out more water-related facts. As nicely illustrated by the diagram on the next page, the United Nations research team concluded that fresh, non-polluted water should be considered one of our most valuable resources. While we are all acutely aware of the vital role water plays in keeping us alive, it wasn't until recently that the world's supply of drinkable water became a concern.

Using numbers put forth by the United Nations, 75 percent of the Earth is covered by water, yet 97.5 percent of that is salt water, which leaves just 2.5 percent as fresh water. However, 70 percent of that is frozen, leaving only 30 percent as ground water that we have access to. Unfortunately, a large amount of *that* water is polluted, so what we are left with as usable non-polluted fresh water is less than 1 percent of the Earth's total. And 70 percent of that 1 percent is primarily used for agriculture animal feed, and another 22 percent for industry. Therefore, what we have remaining is about 0.08 percent for domestic use.[15] Clearly, there is good reason to make a concerted conservation effort when using water around the house by using low-flow showerheads, not letting water run as we brush our teeth, and so on. But by far the most significant impact we can have on our conservation efforts is to reduce agriculture water usage. The 70 percent of non-polluted water that we use to irrigate fields is mostly going to animal feed crops. Not only are we using an inordinate amount of water in the production of animal feed, but upward of 85 percent of that feed is turned out as manure soon after consumption.[16] And that's the next concern. Farmed animals are not much more than a system for converting natural resources into manure, a by-product, which, to add insult to injury, is largely responsible for increasing the amount of water pollution so that our already dwindling supply of usable water becomes still scarcer.

And of course to transport the manure away, well, that takes energy too, from, of course, fossil fuel.

This depiction does not take into account the water damage that livestock contributes to. The livestock sector not only uses a vast amount

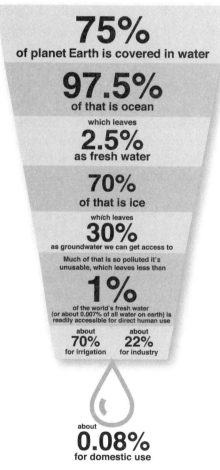

75%
of planet Earth is covered in water

97.5%
of that is ocean

which leaves
2.5%
as fresh water

70%
of that is ice

which leaves
30%
as groundwater we can get access to

Much of that is so polluted it's
unusable, which leaves less than
1%
of the world's fresh water
(or about 0.007% of all water on earth) is
readily accessible for direct human use

about
70%
for irrigation

about
22%
for industry

about
0.08%
for domestic use

Of the usable water we have, most is used to irrigate feed crops for animals, leaving very little water for direct human consumption. (Adapted from the original at treehugger.com. Used with permission.)

of water directly but, according to the United Nations, is responsible for significant water pollution. This is from the executive summary of a U.N. report, speaking of livestock production:

✳ It is probably the largest sectoral source of water pollution, contributing to eutrophication, "dead" zones in coastal areas, degradation of coral reefs, human health problems, emergence of antibiotic resistance and many others. The major sources of pollution are from animal wastes, antibiotics, and hormones, chemicals from tanneries, fertilizers and pesticides used for feedcrops, and sediments from eroded pastures.[17]

Water requirements to produce 1 pound of beef, not taking into consideration the water pollution caused by manure are as follows:

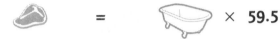

Factoring in irrigation for feed crops, it takes at least 2500 U.S. gallons of water to yield 1 pound of beef[18] (some sources estimate it can take as much as 12,000 gallons[19]). That's 59.5 standard bathtubs' worth of water to get a couple of sirloin steaks or a big helping of prime rib to your table.

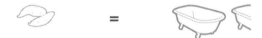

In contrast, only about 60 gallons of water, enough to fill 1.36 bathtubs, are needed to produce a pound of sweet potatoes.[20]

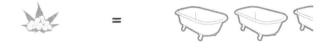

About 100 gallons of water, the capacity of 2.3 standard-size bathtubs, are needed to grow one pound of hemp seed.[21]

In short, the amount of water it takes to produce a pound of beef is 25 times more than needed to grow a pound of hemp seed, and about 42 times more than needed to produce a pound of sweet potatoes.

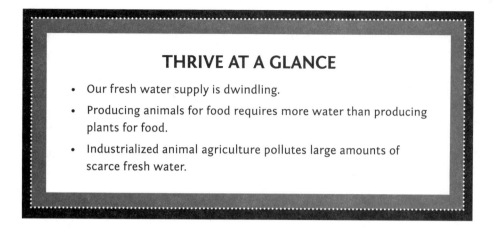

THRIVE AT A GLANCE

- Our fresh water supply is dwindling.
- Producing animals for food requires more water than producing plants for food.
- Industrialized animal agriculture pollutes large amounts of scarce fresh water.

FOSSIL FUEL

Oil, coal, and natural gas are collectively known as fossil fuel and abundantly overused in North America. In fact, 85 percent of energy produced in North America is derived from the burning of these carbon-rich deposits.[22] Essentially, fossil fuel is made up of prehistoric plant matter that, millions of years ago, extracted and "quarantined" carbon from the ancient atmosphere. As with plants today, they were made

> Plants are in fact solidified sunlight and, as such, the energy of the sun will be released back into the atmosphere when these ancient plants are burned or decay.

up of a combination of cellulose and sunlight. A plant is primarily the result of the process of photosynthesis, in which chlorophyll converts sunlight into carbohydrate for the plant to "eat." Cellulose is the plant matter created. Therefore, plants are in fact solidified sunlight and, as such, the energy of the sun will be released back into the atmosphere when these ancient plants are burned or decay. As Thom Hartmann eloquently puts it in his excellent book *The Last Hours of Ancient Sunlight,* fossil fuel is our savings account for the sun's energy that shone on Earth millions of years ago. *All* energy originates from the sun. Plants, of course, cannot exist without sunlight, and animals, of course, cannot exist without plants. We, as humans, are solar-powered too. Eating plants that, through photosynthesis, trap sunlight and use it to fabricate vitamins, grow cellulose, and draw minerals from the soil pass on to us the energy that originated from the sun.

Since our population began to grow considerably, and since our demand for energy paralleled this expansion, we got to a point where we could no longer rely simply on the current sunlight—solidified into trees—as a form of fuel (firewood) to keep pace with our escalating energy needs. So, we had to break open our savings account. Coal was the first of the fossil fuels to be burned since it was easily accessible and needed no refinement. Initially it was used in place of wood as a means to heat a room. The warmth and light from sunlight that had shone down on the Earth millions of years ago, combined with cellulose and carbon dioxide, was now being released back into the atmosphere. Enter the age of artificial climate change.

Soon after came the discovery of oil and the realization that it could serve as a dense source of energy, at that time primarily used for heating. The ability we accrued to refine and utilize it changed our path of evolution. It allowed us to grow our population more rapidly and has led to our ability to sustain its swift growth rate. Since the first chunk of coal was ignited, we have grown ever more dependent on our savings account, primarily consisting of two sources of oil.

The United States gets its oil from Canada and the Middle East. Neither source is without its share of challenges.

The Alberta oil sands, often referred to as the tar sands, supply a vast amount of the world's oil. Canada is now the number-one supplier of oil—ahead of Saudi Arabia—to the United States.[23]

The rich carbon deposits found in the oil sands are in the form of a thick, heavy type of oil called bitumen. Geologically, bitumen has not been "cooked" long enough to reach the light viscosity of coveted Middle Eastern crude.

The energy required to take bitumen from the earth and transform it into usable carbon products is extraordinary. In fact, some estimates suggest that for every unity of energy we obtain from the oil sands, we have used an equal amount of energy to extract and process it.[24] And since that energy comes from the burning of fossil fuel, our net energy gain would be zero. Clearly, this cancels out the oil sands as a solution to our energy shortfall. In addition, for every barrel of oil extracted and processed, three times that amount of water is needed, 90 percent of which is then deemed polluted.[25]

But the oil sands are great for the economy. Within our current structure, inefficiency is at the root of a robust economic system. The more people we can put to work doing things—and being paid well for it—the better. Alberta leads the way; it is the only Canadian province with a monetary surplus, so the argument is that that province must be doing something right. Or is it inefficient?

The crude oil imported from the Middle East is much easier to extract from the earth and therefore takes much less energy and involves a less labor-intensive process. Plus, turning it into a usable product, such as gasoline, is considerably less involved, so that the process again requires less energy to be burned and fewer hands to make it happen.

There are clearly issues with both sources of oil. While less energy is required to extract and process crude oil form the Middle East, it must be transported to North America to be of use. As you can imagine, an immense amount of energy must be spent to load millions of gallons of oil on a freighter and have it shipped thousands of miles to North America. Also, it is not desirable that the United States be dependent on Middle Eastern nations for its energy, since its relationship with some of these nations is tumultuous. Should those nations decide to "turn off the tap," they would bring the United States, at its current rate of oil consumption, to its knees within a month.

Energy independence starts with reduced demand. And being more efficient is something we can all begin immediately. From there, new energy solutions can be developed domestically to sever our reliance on foreign oil.

And then there's the question of remaining supply. "How much more oil is left?" With deposits to our energy savings account being made only every few million years, how long can we continue to spend without earning before we're broke?

That's exactly the question being asked by many prominent scientists, many of whom subscribe to the "peak oil" theory. Defined as "the point at which maximum global oil production is reached, after which the rate of production goes into terminal decline," the "peak oil" hypothesis has become widely accepted.[26] Most who study the subject agree that the Earth will at some point simply run out of oil. But when exactly that time will come is hotly debated. Many scientists who study the subject believe we are on the cusp of peak oil now, or may have already experienced it, dating the start of the decline around 2009. But even the optimistic peak oil theorists warn that the peak is *likely* to happen within our generation, beginning in 2020. From there, as peak oil believers point out, a steep and terminal decline will abruptly follow.

A minority within the scientific community feels the decline will occur much later. If we were to run out of oil, they theorize, it would be centuries, or even millennia, from now. At which point, according to this minority, it is assumed that by then we'll have developed the technology to harness alternative forms of energy from the sun, wind, and the ever-changing sea tide.

ASSUMED.

But I think it's safe to say that no one really knows when that point will be. Or, as some see it, if it will come at all.

I should point out that there are in fact a handful of prominent scientists who dismiss the peak oil theory altogether. These people, subscribers to the abiotic hypothesis, as it is called, believe oil regenerates itself more quickly than what is classically believed, because, they theorize, it's not actually fossil fuel at all.[27] Therefore, it is not subject to the multi-million-year process of turning ancient decaying plants and dinosaurs into crude. The abiotic hypothesis posits that oil is a natural product produced in the mantel of the Earth. Therefore, as the theory goes, millions of years are not needed to create oil; the Earth manufactures and spews it out in a timely fashion.

> Since the combustion of oil creates toxic gas and releases pollution into the air that significantly increases the risk of disease, the less oil we need to burn, the better off we'll be.

So let's assume, against the vast scientific majority, that we will not reach peak oil in our generation—and maybe never. There's still an undeniable problem with our level of oil consumption: emissions. Best known as greenhouse gases, these emissions are being blamed for some pretty big problems. And some observers (the United Nations, for example) suggest those emissions are what cause climate change. (I expand on this topic in the "Air Quality" section on page 50.)

(What a joke... "Carbon footprint.")

Regardless, I think we can all agree that, since the combustion of oil creates toxic gas and releases pollution into the air that significantly increases the risk of disease (including cardiovascular disease),[28] the less oil we need to burn, the better off we'll be.

Ha. HA. YES.

As humans, we obtain our energy from food, which we produce by burning fossil fuel. So, essentially, we are trading the stored energy of fossil fuel (which originated from the sun) for caloric energy that's of biological use to us.

And each time we do this, as with any energy transfer, there is a loss. But when we pass that energy through an animal, the loss becomes significantly greater.

Growing food to feed to animals, which will in turn feed us, requires significantly more arable land than growing plants for our direct consumption. The reason so much food needs to be grown to feed these animals is that very little of the food energy passed on to the livestock is returned through their meat.

To give an idea of how energy is lost in the production of animals, here's a breakdown:

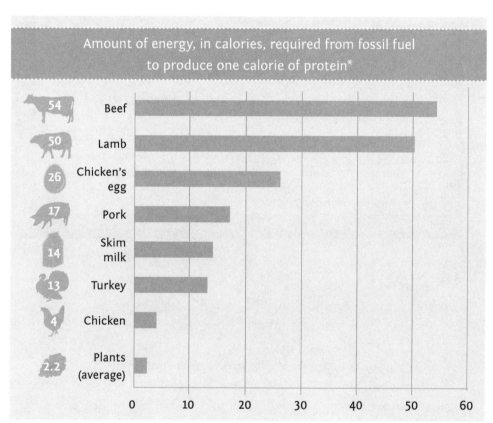

Amount of energy, in calories, required from fossil fuel to produce one calorie of protein*

	Calories
54 Beef	
50 Lamb	
26 Chicken's egg	
17 Pork	
14 Skim milk	
13 Turkey	
4 Chicken	
2.2 Plants (average)	

On average, in the United States it takes 25.4 calories of fossil fuel energy to yield one calorie of animal protein for human consumption.[29]

In contrast, to obtain one calorie from plant-based protein, 2.2 calories of fossil fuel need to be burned.[30] This figure takes in account all fuel expenditures, including the energy it takes to produce fertilizer to grow the food and to run the farm machinery that harvests it.

Source of data: Cornell Science News, "U.S. Could Feed 800 Million People with Grain that Livestock Eat ..."[31]

*Of course, meat is inherently higher in protein than plants, so to make this comparison fairer, I've compared only the calories from protein. Contrasting the total number of calories produced from animal sources and those produced from plant sources would give an even more dramatically lopsided picture.

AIR QUALITY

When it's burned, fossil fuel provides us with energy by releasing stored heat and light from "ancient sunlight." However, along with the release of energy from prehistoric rays of sun comes the unwelcome by-product of sequestered carbon from prehistory, known as emissions. As dinosaurs and other ancient animals exhaled, plants collected their wayward carbon dioxide and over millions of years reduced it to fossilized sludge, which we know as coal and oil. When we burn coal and oil, the combustion releases this long-quarantined and ancient animal breath into our modern world. Believe it or not, each time you start your car, the emissions from the tailpipe are, in part, dinosaur breath being set free.

While plants may consume carbon dioxide, it's poisonous to us oxygen-breathing creatures. And because of this, reducing the amount of emissions set free into our atmosphere is in our best interest. Besides being deadly to inhale, carbon dioxide and other greenhouse gas emissions are being blamed for one of the most feared threats of modern times: artificial climate change. While most scientists agree that the Earth has experienced, and will continue to experience, a natural fluctuation in temperature change, a growing body of evidence suggests that emissions created by the combustion of fossil fuel—known as greenhouse gases—are playing a significant role in manipulating this cycle. Commonly referred to as global warming, the average temperature of the Earth is continuing to rise.

As the sun's warm rays shine on the Earth, some of their heat is absorbed, while some is reflected back into the atmosphere, escaping into space. However, greenhouse gases trap atmospheric heat from the sun's rays within the Earth's atmosphere, thereby causing temperature on Earth to rise. This is aptly known as the greenhouse effect. As the amount of greenhouse gases increases, so too does the average temperature of the Earth. Even a small temperature change can have a profound negative effect on ecosystems. And there have been significant changes already.

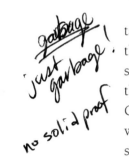

Former U.S. vice president Al Gore's 2006 Oscar-winning documentary, _An Inconvenient Truth,_ shone a spotlight on the human hastening of this dire phenomenon. Citing evidence from the leading scientists on the subject, the film put forth the hypothesis that we are indeed to blame for the rapidly increasing average temperature rise of the Earth's atmosphere. Corroborated by a glut of scientific heavy-hitters, the film captured the world's attention and in doing so sounded the alarm bell. Its message was simple: we are to blame and we must change our ways before it's too late.

In one of the most compelling scenes of the film, computer-generated images showed areas, such as Florida, Shanghai, Calcutta, and Manhattan, slipping beneath the ocean surface as the polar ice caps melted because of an increase in global temperature, causing sea levels to rise. According to the film, if we continue on our current path, the polar ice caps will melt enough "in the near future" to cause a 20-foot rise in sea level, which would trigger the destruction of major coastal cities and result in "one hundred million environmental refugees."

> The volume of emissions created by operating cars, trucks, buses, airplanes, and ships, while considerable, pales in comparison to the volume of CO_2-equivalent greenhouse gases released through raising animals for food.

The film blamed our seemingly insatiable thirst for energy. Required to fuel our modern lifestyle and derived from burning fossil fuel, our energy needs and "wants" create emissions. A lot of emissions. And as a result an extraordinary amount of greenhouse gases are produced. *Everything* we do requires energy. And almost all of it is obtained by the burning of fossil fuel.

While the film certainly captured the world's attention, it drew criticism for offering few solutions to a problem it so passionately described. Adamantly making a case for human-hastened climate change and impending global disaster as a consequence, it left many feeling helpless. Other than suggesting, "Drive hybrid cars and replace incandescent light bulbs with compact fluorescents," the film left viewers wanting to know how they could mitigate the part they might be playing in the advancement of the crisis.

Coincidentally, also in 2006, a United Nations report was released stating that animal agriculture is one of the greatest contributing factors to anthropologic climate change because of its inordinate energy demands. The report went on to say that animal agriculture is a larger producer of greenhouse gas emissions, and therefore a larger contributor to artificial climate change, than all modes of transportation. *Combined.* The volume of emissions created by operating cars, trucks, buses, airplanes, and ships, while considerable, pales in comparison to the volume of CO_2-equivalent greenhouse gases released through raising animals for food. According to the U.N. report, *Livestock's Long Shadow,* a whopping 18 percent of these emissions result from raising livestock for food. In comparison, 13 percent of total greenhouse gas emissions (measured in CO_2 equivalent) can be attributed to the transportation sector.[32] As you can imagine, when the information was released that raising animals for food created 5 percent more greenhouse gas emissions than did all of transportation, people were in a state of disbelief.

Those best-intentioned carpooling hybrid drivers who stopped at the drive-thru to pick up their daily ham and egg sandwiches were caught off guard. Now there was confusion.

Here's the reason: greenhouse gas emissions comprise three types of gases: CO_2 (carbon dioxide), nitrous oxide, and methane. While CO_2 is the most common in terms of volume (it's what's expelled from a car's exhaust pipe), its global warming potential, or GWP, is 23 times lower than that of methane.[33] Emitted primarily from ruminants, most notably cows, methane has been fingered by the United Nations as a major contributor to anthropologic climate change. When cows and other ruminants eat grass, their digestive system breaks it down, mechanically, through chewing, and chemically, through fermentation. And a natural by-product of fermentation is gas, in this case, methane.

Yet, even worse, the vast majority of cows in North America are "produced" in factory farms where grass is not on the menu. Wheat, corn, and soy are popular feed choices since they "encourage" cows to reach their slaughter weight sooner. Cows have four stomachs, designed for the assimilation of grass, so when cows eat wheat, corn, and soy, digestive issues "erupt." And as a direct result, excessive gas is created and released into the atmosphere, contributing to the containment of atmospheric heat. And then there's the manure. Nitrous oxide has a global warming potential 296 times greater than that of CO_2, and 65 percent of the world's nitrous oxide emanates from livestock manure.[34]

So, clearly, the greatest single thing we can do as individuals to reduce the amount of greenhouse gases we contribute to producing is to eat foods that create fewer emissions in their production.

But what about those who dismiss the theory that we humans (and our farmed animals) have anything to do with climate change? Those who believe that the Earth is going through a natural cycle and we are just along for the ride and are in no way responsible for the average warming of the Earth? They are going against the overwhelming scientific majority and contradicting the findings by United Nations scientists, but to be fair, there is still a small scientific community that doesn't believe we are to blame, at all.

However, even if this small group of scientists turns out to be spot on, this is undeniable: when fossil fuel (and oil, if it turns out not to be fossil fuel after all) is converted into energy, it must be burned. And burning fossil fuel creates toxic gases, most commonly referred to as pollution.[35] And there's a direct correlation between air pollution levels and mortality rates.

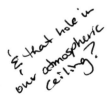

Beginning in 1974, researchers at Harvard University set out to conduct a long-term study in hopes of revealing the correlation between air pollution and our number-one killer, cardiovascular disease. It had long been thought that air pollution could not be a good thing, but a long-term study on its health effects hadn't yet been conducted. And while we knew that the lack of minerals in our food is a major contributing risk factor for CVD, what about the microscopic particulates that we breathe in—air pollution? For this investigation, known as the Six Cities Study, the researchers collected data—over the course of 14 to 16 years—on 8000 people. The results showed what a rational person might suspect; that the greater amount of pollution in the air, the greater the risk of death from cardiovascular disease.[36] But the unmistakable correlation between the *amount* of air pollution and the cardiovascular disease mortality rates was striking.

> The pollution in rural areas is generally created by food production.

The researchers concluded that there was a clear connection.

While it's true that most of the thick layer of pollution over the cities is attributable to automobiles, the pollution in rural areas is generally created by food production. Fewer people live in those areas, so perhaps, we might think, fewer people are directly affected by the pollution, but this is also the geographical space where our food is grown. As we know, plants quarantine carbon dioxide. When those plants are food crops, having them take in pollution becomes a problem. The pollution literally becomes part of our food. And then us.

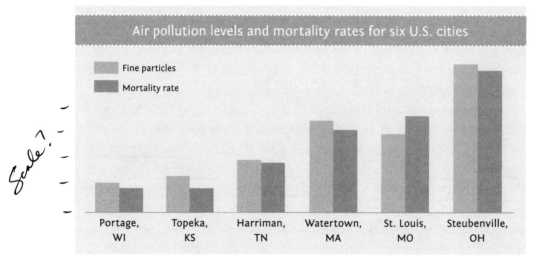

Air pollution levels and mortality rates for six U.S. cities

Fine particles
Mortality rate

Portage, WI   Topeka, KS   Harriman, TN   Watertown, MA   St. Louis, MO   Steubenville, OH

Scale?

As you can see, the correlation between pollution and risk of death from CVD is striking.

Data adapted from Harvard Six Cities Study.

WHAT ABOUT EATING LOCAL TO REDUCE EMISSIONS?

Eating food that's been produced locally—commonly understood to be within a 100-mile radius—makes sense. Logically, the less distance food needs to travel to reach those who will consume it, the fewer emissions will be created.

In fact, this simple concept began gaining acceptance, and then even popularity, in 2005. Some early adopters were hailing it as our solution to climate change by reducing those dreaded "food miles" (the distance food must be transported from producer to consumer).

The thought of air-shipping food all over the world—bananas from Ecuador, pineapple from Hawaii, coconut from Thailand—seemed excessively decadent. Food miles were mounting, adding hundreds of thousands of pounds of CO_2 emissions to our atmosphere each year. But what was most disconcerting to those making an effort to eat local was our desire for out-of-season fruit—pears from Australia, peaches from South America, grapes from Chile—that, if we were patient, could be obtained locally in a few months.

Several books were published on the subject and, as the movement continued to progress, pop culture embraced it.

In fact, the word "locavore" was coined to describe proponents of the movement, and in 2007 the term not only made its way into the *New Oxford American Dictionary* but was named that dictionary's "word of the year."[37] The dictionary defined *locavore* simply as "a person who endeavors to eat only locally produced food." The locavores had arrived.

Awesome!

While I subscribe to the concept, grow a bunch of my own food, and shop at farmers' markets weekly, I couldn't help but wonder: of all the greenhouse gas emissions created by the production and delivery of food, how much of those were as a result of transportation (food miles) as opposed to production? Well, as I found out, I wasn't the only one with this question. Thankfully, some of those who shared my curiosity happened to be research scientists at Carnegie Mellon University in Pittsburgh. And with the means to get an answer, Christopher L. Weber and H. Scott Matthews conducted a study to determine the actual amount of CO_2-equivalent gases emitted by transportation of food, compared to the amount emitted by its production. The results were fascinating. Weber and Matthews published their findings in the prestigious journal *Environmental Science & Technology.*[38]

In the report the authors state, "Our analysis shows that despite all the attention given to food miles, the distance that food travels only accounts for around 11 percent of the average American household's food-related greenhouse gas emissions, while production contributes to 83 percent." A significant divide to say the least: 7.5 times more greenhouse gas emissions are created in the production of food than by its delivery. Specifically, nitrous oxide and methane, inadvertently produced by fertilizers (for animal feed crops), manure, and gas expelled during the animals' digestion account for a large portion of the CO_2-equivalent gases created during production.[39]

> 7.5 times more greenhouse gas emissions are created in the production of food than by its delivery.

The findings shed light on what many others and I had suspected: while eating local is sensible, environmentally speaking, *what* we eat is of greater importance. Significantly greater importance.

THE GREATEST EMISSION CREATOR

In July 2007, the compelling results of a study conducted by a team at the National Institute of Livestock and Grassland Science in Tsukuba, Japan, were published, and reported on in the U.K. press.[40] *New Scientist* magazine immediately picked up the story, and within hours the hard-to-believe numbers had gripped the scientific community's attention.[41] The study found that, when all factors were taken into consideration, the amount of greenhouse gases released into the atmosphere from the production of 2.2 pounds of beef was the equivalent of 80.08 pounds of carbon dioxide. To put that latter figure into perspective, it's the equivalent in CO_2 emissions of a midsize car that gets 26 miles to the gallon being driven 160 miles.

According to the U.S. Department of Agriculture, the average Canadian eats about 68.4 pounds of beef per year.[42] The CO_2 equivalent from its production would be equal to roadtripping in a midsize car from Vancouver to Toronto, and 90 percent of the way back: a total distance of 4976 miles.

The U.S. numbers are even higher, considering the average American eats 96.4 pounds of beef per year.[43] Producing that beef would create

1595 kilograms of CO_2, which equates to driving 7008 miles, or a road trip from New York City to Los Angeles *and* back, and then one-way from NYC to Miami. That's one person, for one year.

Not that this is at all realistic, but what *if* everyone in the United States stopped eating beef for one year? With a population of 307 million, the savings in CO_2 equivalent would be the same as what would be conserved by not driving that midsize car the distance of over 2 trillion miles (2,151,501,902,400, to be exact). Considerable, to say the least. And, in fact, since the average distance to the moon is 238,857 miles,[44] if everyone in the U.S. stopped eating beef for one year, that would be like not driving a distance equivalent to 9,007,489 trips to the moon. Think about it: the driving distance of over 9 *million* trips to the moon.

> If everyone in the U.S. stopped eating beef for one year, that would be like not driving a distance equivalent to 9,007,489 trips to the moon.

HA. HA.

And if Canadians abstained from eating beef for one year? We'd save in emissions as much as if we'd chosen to not drive our cars a distance equal to 693,961 trips to the moon.

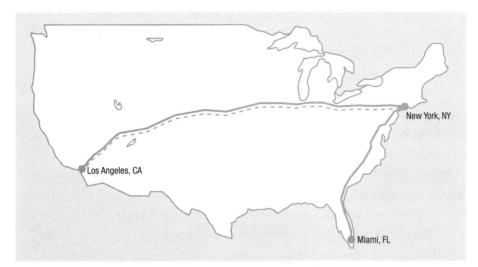

Driving equivalent in CO_2-equivalent savings if the average American did not eat factory-farmed beef for one year.

The same study also noted that the energy needed to produce the amount of fertilizer required to grow the feed to be consumed by that cattle is significant. For each kilogram of beef, 160 megajoules of energy is burned in fertilizer production. That's the same amount of energy that would be used to light a 100-watt bulb for 20 days.

So, to produce enough beef for the average Canadian to consume in one year would require the same amount of energy as keeping one 100-watt bulb lit for 622 days, or 14,928 hours.

By not eating beef for a year, an average American would conserve enough energy to light the bulb for 876 days.

Cows are not the only problem. According to a U.K. government agency called the Department for the Environment, Food and Rural Affairs (or DEFRA), while ruminants, such as cows and sheep, produce the most methane, other animals are not completely free from blame. The agency states that for every unit of meat from a pig that's produced, five times that amount of greenhouse gas is released into the atmosphere. For chickens, it's four times.[45] So while ruminants are the greatest offenders, energy inefficiency, and therefore excessive emission production, is a factor in raising all livestock. While raising chickens produces less CO_2 emissions than raising any other farmed animals, the level of emissions is still double that of even the most inefficient plant crops.

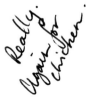

For every one pound of chicken produced, four pounds of CO_2-equivalent emissions is released.[46] Therefore, the production of about 2.2 pounds of chicken releases as much CO_2-equivalent emissions as driving 14.6 miles.

Since the average amount of chicken eaten per person in Canada is 66.22 pounds[47] and for every pound of chicken produced four pounds of carbon dioxide is released into the atmosphere, that would add an annual amount of carbon dioxide to the atmosphere equivalent to the emissions from a midsize car being driven 439.4 miles (the distance from Prince George to Calgary).

And for Americans it's worse since they eat, on average, 102.3 pounds of chicken meat per year,[48] contributing 409.2 pounds of carbon dioxide into the atmosphere—the equivalent of driving 679 miles (the distance from Chicago to Washington, D.C.).

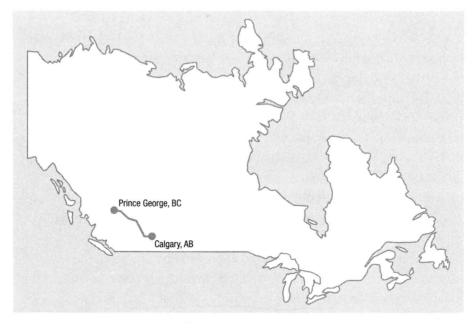

Driving equivalent in CO$_2$-equivalent savings if the average Canadian did not eat chicken for one year.

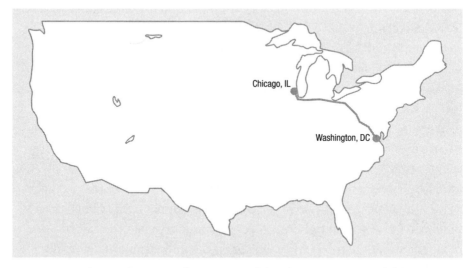

Driving equivalent in CO$_2$-equivalent savings if the average American did not eat chicken for one year.

As for pork?

Since for every 2.2 pounds of pork produced, about 11 pounds of carbon dioxide is released, that's the same amount of CO_2-equivalent emissions as driving 18.25 miles.

Therefore, because of the average Canadian's annual pork consumption of 50.49 pounds,[49] 114.5 pounds of CO_2-equivalent emissions would be released into the atmosphere. This works out to the equivalent of driving 418 miles, about the distance from Saskatoon to Lethbridge.

The average American eats 62.25 pounds of pork per year,[50] its production releasing 148 pounds of CO_2-equivalent emissions, which translates into what would be emitted driving 540.2 miles, about the distance from Pittsburgh to Providence, Rhode Island.

As more reports were conducted and as studies emerged, the inordinate amount of emissions created by livestock become an article of public knowledge (among the informed public, at least). And as such, concerned citizens begin wisely looking for ways they could be part of the solution. Those seeking to mitigate climate change and address other issues surrounding emission production began entertaining creative ways to do so.

In August 2007, *The Sunday Times* newspaper in the United Kingdom ran an article with the headline: "Walking to the shops damages planet more than going by car."[51] As we can assume was the intent, it captured attention. The article, penned by a staff writer, consisted of an interview with Chris Goodall, author of *How to Live a Low-Carbon Life*. Quoting Mr. Goodall's book, the article stated that based on official government fuel emission figures, about two pounds of carbon dioxide would be released into the atmosphere by driving a typical U.K. car three miles. In comparison, walking three miles would burn about 180 calories. If those calories were obtained by eating beef, the emissions associated with its production would come in at about 7.9 pounds, nearly four times as much as the emissions from driving the car. What about obtaining the calories from milk? It would take about 1¾ cups of milk to match the caloric requirements of the three-mile walk. So, if the milk came from a modern dairy farm, 2.6 pounds of carbon dioxide would be released, which is 25 percent more than would be released by the journey by car.

And as you may imagine, this article garnered attention, most of it from those who mistakenly assumed Chris was advocating we forgo

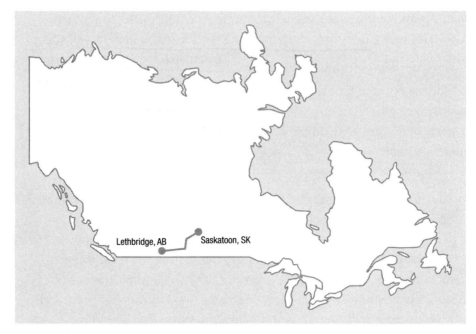

Driving equivalent in CO₂-equivalent savings if the average Canadian did not eat pork for one year.

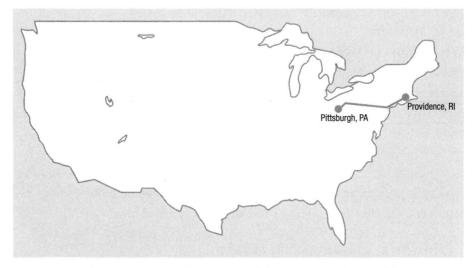

Driving equivalent in CO₂-equivalent savings if the average American did not eat pork for one year.

walking and increase our use of the automobile. Of course, this wasn't Goodall's point. By simply drawing our attention to the fact that all energy originates somewhere else, in my opinion, Goodall powerfully made his point: nothing is free. Even if we "generate" the energy ourselves, it had to come from somewhere, in his examples, from food. And, as we know, food production is a major energy draw. What I appreciate about this example is its articulation of energy origin, transfer, and use.

> A food source that emits fewer emissions during its life cycle is a good start for a more environmentally friendly food choice.

Of course, there are several factors not addressed in his example. How fit was the person? As we know, the fitter the person, the fewer calories he or she will burn, since a trait of greater fitness is improved efficiency. As efficiency improves, the fuel requirements (food in this case) to travel a given distance will decline. And by how much did this fictitious person reduce his or her risk of osteoporosis, type 2 diabetes, and cardiovascular disease by walking to the store? And what about the significant amount of energy used to manufacture the car? But that wasn't the point.

Certainly Chris Goodall did an excellent job in communicating his point in a "sticky" manner that started a discussion.

WHAT CONSTITUTES ENVIRONMENTALLY FRIENDLY FOOD CHOICES?

Obviously, simply not eating isn't a viable long-term solution. Clearly, a food source that emits fewer emissions during its life cycle is a good start for a more environmentally friendly food choice. And one that isn't a land, water, and fossil-fuel hog would be nice too.

In 2008 my colleagues and I at Sequel Naturals enlisted the help of a Calgary-based company called Conscious Brands to determine the best food options from an environmental perspective. Focusing on breakfast, the report considered the following three different types of breakfasts:

TRADITIONAL AMERICAN BREAKFAST

Consisting of two eggs, two slices of bacon, two links of sausage, one slice of toast, and 5.3 ounces of hash browns, the traditional breakfast scored 2.9 pounds of carbon dioxide.

LIGHT AMERICAN BREAKFAST

The light American breakfast comprised ½ cup of cereal, 1 cup of cow's milk, 1 cup of yogurt, and half a banana; it came in considerably lower, at just 12.3 ounces of carbon dioxide.

✳PLANT-BASED WHOLE FOOD SMOOTHIE BREAKFAST

The fully plant-based smoothie option, made up of a dry weight of 2.3 ounces of hemp protein, yellow pea protein, brown rice protein, flaxseed, maca, and chlorella came in at only 1.2 ounces of carbon dioxide. That's 10 times fewer emissions than that of the light American breakfast, and 38 times fewer than the traditional American breakfast. If we wanted to blend the smoothie with half a banana, it would come in at 2.1 ounces, still 22 times lower than the traditional American breakfast, and 5.8 times lower than the light American breakfast.[52]

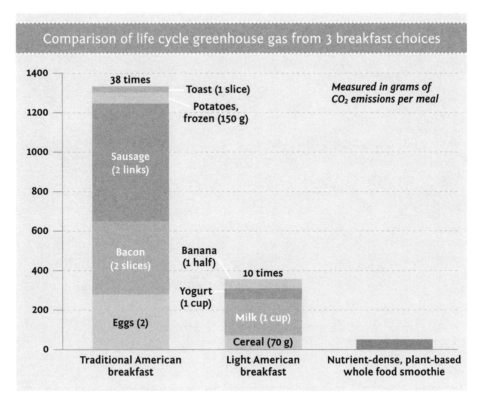

CO$_2$-equivalent emissions comparison between breakfast options.

So, with these numbers in hand, we can consider some options. For example, if one person were to switch his or her traditional American breakfast for a plant-based whole food option, the CO_2-equivalent savings would be equal to driving a midsize car from Vancouver, B.C., to Tijuana, Mexico: the whole length of the Western United States.[53]

Now, if everyone in the United States swapped his or her traditional breakfast for the plant-based option, the amount of emissions saved would be the equivalent to those created driving over 409 billion miles (409,853,744,250 miles, to be exact). That's equal in distance to over 1.7 million trips to the moon.

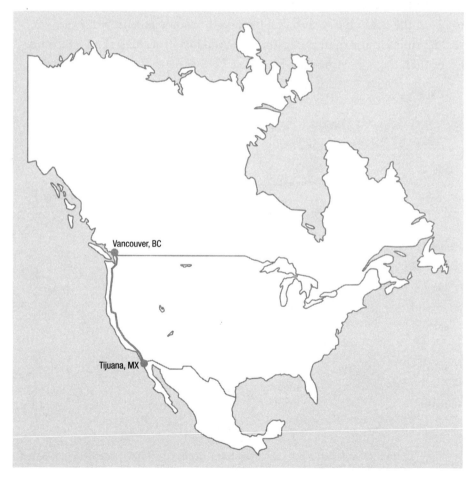

Driving equivalent of CO_2-equivalent savings if the average American swapped his or her traditional American breakfast option for a plant-based smoothie for one year.

In reality, not everyone in the United States eats a traditional American breakfast. Some eat lighter. Some eat heavier. But even if we use the light American breakfast and compare it to the greatly more nutritious plant-based option, the emission savings is impressive. In fact, it's with this information that we were able to fine tune my Vega Complete Whole Food Health Optimizer blender drink formula so that its production would require the least amount of each natural resource (more information on page 342).

This report was all very encouraging to me. It nicely illustrated that even though a substantial amount of natural resources are spent in obtaining our required nutrition, each of us has the ability to measurably reduce environmental strain by simply making informed food choices. *What we eat is paramount.*

But simply spending natural resources—and incurring the environment's cost associated with their use—is not the only consideration when selecting food. As I discussed in detail in Chapter 1, micronutrients are the most valuable component when assessing a food's nutritional worth.

And realizing that an inordinate amount of natural resources are required to produce food in this country, as well as appreciating the bearing on overall health that micronutrients have, I grew curious to see if there was a system that took both related issues into account when producing food, a system with a simple mandate: gain the highest levels of each micronutrient, expend the fewest resources to do so. I couldn't find one. In my search I did, however, come across carbon labeling—the displaying of a given food product's CO_2-equivalent emissions during its life cycle—and I did find an unrelated nutrient labeling system that indicated the nutrient density of select foods. But I found nothing that worked in concert to marry the two. This seemed to me to be a blind spot. A blind spot with ubiquitous, varied, and expensive consequences: excessive soil depletion, extreme fresh water consumption, fossil fuel gluttony, exorbitant greenhouse gases belching, to name just a few of the environmental issues. The

> ✱ If we knew that a food company was using less of each natural resource to produce more nutrient-dense food, we could, appreciating the importance of this, then choose to "vote" for that company by buying its products.

health issues associated with this blind spot were also rampant: constant hunger; overeating co-existing with malnourishment; general fatigue, difficulty sleeping, and dependence on stimulants, such as coffee and refined sugar; as well as significantly increased risk for many diseases, including cardiovascular disease. Could the solution be a simple ratio displayed on food labels, one part the amount of each natural resource expended, one part the micronutrients within the food that are gained in return? I believe that such a label would add another layer of transparency and completeness to the food system as a whole. It would clearly give us, as consumers, vital information upon which to base our buying decisions. If we knew that a food company was using less of each natural resource to produce more nutrient-dense food, we could, appreciating the importance of this, then choose to "vote" for that company by buying its products. And of course, in doing so, we would facilitate its growth, based on our values aligning with its values.

Values. ☺

THRIVE AT A GLANCE

- The burning of fossil fuel releases CO_2 into the atmosphere.

- It's commonly accepted by experts that climate change is a result of too much CO_2 and CO_2e in the atmosphere.

- Due to inefficiency, animal agriculture requires that many times more fossil fuel be burned (and CO_2 be released) than for the farming of plants.

- Excess CO_2 in the atmosphere has been linked to higher levels of heart conditions such as cardiovascular disease.

- CO_2e greenhouse gasses such as methane and nitrous oxide emitted from animals (and animal waste) have a Global Warming Potential many times greater than that of CO_2.

- The inefficient production of food is a far greater producer of CO_2e than the transportation of food.

- More CO_2e is released into the atmosphere as a result of animal agriculture than by all of transportation, combined.

- For the average American, switching to a plant-based diet would prevent more CO_2e from being released into the atmosphere than by eliminating driving altogether.

AN APPETITE FOR CHANGE:
Environmental and Health Solutions Through Food

3

As you've read in earlier chapters, when we factor in the natural resources required in their production, some foods are easier on the environment than others, and some stand out as exceptionally resource-intensive to produce.

As you'll read below, the Carbon Trust in the United Kingdom has introduced carbon labels to help British consumers understand the environmental implications of their food selections. The labels inform them as to how much carbon they will be responsible for "emitting" if they choose to buy certain foods.

Yay U.K.!

That information's important, but it's only half of the equation.

Since micronutrients are the true measure of a food's value, in this chapter I look at ways to gain the most micronutrients while expending the fewest natural resources. I've put together a system that takes both environmental strain *and* micronutrient yield into consideration; I call it the "nutrient-to-resources ratio," and will explain it in detail later in the chapter. Foods with the highest nutrient-to-resources ratio are therefore the ones I suggest become the base of our diet, not only for peak health but also to put the least amount of strain on our natural resources.

I also compare the monetary cost of different foods. While it's undoubtedly less expensive to gain calories from highly processed food (and food-like substances) than from natural whole food, does the argument that "it's too expensive to eat healthy" hold up when we assess the cost of nutrition (micronutrients) as opposed to calories? How much highly refined food would we have to consume to match the nutrition we could get from a small amount of food in its natural state, and what would the cost difference be?

THE U.K.'S LOW CARBON DIET

In March 2007 the British government put forward a draft bill called the Climate Chage Bill, which stated that the countries of the United Kingdom would be required to reduce their carbon emissions by 80 percent (based on 1990 standards) by the year 2050.[1]

A bold move and, as you might expect, a heavily criticized one by some industries. But despite the expected opposition, the bill was passed in November 2008, becoming law and fueling hopes that Britain would evolve into a low-carbon economy. The United Kingdom was now the only country in the world to have imposed such a law upon itself. But whether its ambitions will be fulfilled ultimately rests upon the actions of its people. Britons have responded to the challenge and, according to polls conducted, are actively seeking ways to reduce their carbon output. Through U.N. reports, most notably *Livestock's Long Shadow*, the British population has responded to the message that the most significant difference an individual can make is by way of informed food choices.

Industry's response to consumer concern was swift. Playing to consumers' interest (that could perhaps ultimately become a market demand), a nonprofit company called the Carbon Trust sprang up. Targeting companies wanting to establish a "carbon footprint" for their products, the Carbon Trust offered a CO_2-assessment service and a label to indicate corporate environmental stewardship. Measuring the carbon dioxide emitted during

> *Interesting*
>
> With the aid of the labels, each person can now establish his or her individual "carbon budget," which presumably will make it easier for that individual to stay on a low-carbon diet.

the life cycle (farming, manufacturing, packaging, distribution, and disposal) of a given product, the Carbon Trust offered suggestions as to how carbon dioxide emissions could be reduced, and then would grant a carbon footprint label based on the current carbon dioxide production during the life cycle of the product. The company would make the label part of its packaging. Total "cradle to grave" emissions, measured in grams of CO_2e (carbon dioxide equivalent) emitted as a result of the product and packaging life cycle, were put in plain view.[2]

Further, to meet the Climate Change Bill's target of an 80 percent CO_2-emission reduction by 2050, each individual, says the Carbon Trust, must produce no more (on average) than 8.3 tons of CO_2e per year—which equates to 50 pounds per day. Of that 50 pounds, it's suggested that each person keep the emissions total from his or her food down to no more than 6.5 pounds of CO_2e per day. But wait—what? Clearly, these are abstract numbers, and without a context they have no value. However, thanks to the Carbon Trust, these otherwise unrelatable numbers are put into perspective and given relevance for the average person. With the aid of the labels, each person can now establish his or her individual "carbon budget," which presumably will make it easier for that individual to stay on a low-carbon diet. For example, Tesco, a large grocery store chain in the United Kingdom, enlisted the services of the Carbon Trust to help give its customers a sense of the CO_2-equivalent emissions they might release into the atmosphere should they use particular food products. Its house brand of orange juice, for example, displays a label stating that the production of a one-cup serving of the juice will be directly responsible for releasing 12.5 ounces of carbon dioxide emissions throughout its life cycle.[3] The idea is that with the labeling, those British citizens mindful of their carbon diet will be able to determine if they want to "spend" their limited carbon points to indulge in a glass of orange juice. (By the way, and interesting to note, since carbon labeling is not in itself law in the United Kingdom, only manufacturers of plant-based foods are taking part. That isn't surprising, since products containing meat and dairy would score horribly and presumably scare off those aspiring to stay carbon-lean. The carbon labeling would lift the veil of inefficiency and sales of those products with higher carbon footprints would, presumably, fall.)

I unequivocally commend the proactive stance the U.K. government has taken. However, the assessment services and carbon label of the Carbon Trust, though a step in the right direction, speaks to emissions with no reference to land, water, or fuel consumption. Its main shortcoming is that the emissions score is in no way tied to the nutritional component of the food on which it's affixed. What health-boosting nutrients do we get for our carbon expenditure? How do we decide if we want to "spend" our carbon on food when what we gain in return is not revealed?

To produce our food, we've clearly gone on a resource-spending binge. And, in the haze of our indulgence, what we seek in return has become unclear.

Since the inefficiency of translating natural resources into food has become strikingly apparent, the goal of conscientious food scientists has become to reap more calories from the land while expending fewer resources in doing so. And while I appreciate their effort to maximize return on natural resources' expenditure in food production, I don't feel the calorie is the best point of reference. A calorie is, indeed, a measure of food energy, so at first glance it may seem logical, when converting a precious unit of fossil fuel energy into food energy, to go for the highest possible yield of calories. But as I mentioned in Chapter 1, it's not a lack of calories that makes us sick. In fact, it's quite the opposite. Though the food-producing community may be conscientiously trying to reap more calories from the land for ostensibly environmental reasons, I believe that the health community has valuable insight to share regarding what, specifically, we ought to strive to pull—nutritionally speaking—from the land. And that is nutrient density. As I described in Chapter 1, nutrient density is expressed by a ratio of micronutrients delivered to calories consumed, and the higher the micronutrients and the lower the calories, the better. Nutrient density is a simple and effective way to rate true nutritional value. The goal, for the sake of North Americans' health, should be to draw more micronutrients from our land, not more calories. This rebalance would play a major role in preventing disease and obesity. The odd paradox of modern food production that enables us to be both overfed and undernourished would be immediately eradicated.

But is this what our gov't wants? Is there $ in this?

WHOLE FOODS MARKET: "HEALTH STARTS HERE" PROGRAM

In the spring of 2007, I had the opportunity to spend a long weekend at John Mackey's ranch. Just outside of Austin, Texas, about 40 like-minded people from the natural food industry converged on the Whole Foods Market CEO and visionary's 780-acre ranch. At this event, billed as sports weekend, it didn't take long to gather that Mackey wasn't a typical CEO. Sharing my view of food, John made it clear that he, too, strongly believed that we could lower our rate of disease and health problems in North America simply by making informed food choices.

And because of that simple preventative medicine philosophy, Whole Foods Market has taken the lead in North America by creating a program called "Health Starts Here."[4] As one of the program's proactive measures, nutrient density scores for almost all of its produce were displayed. Initiated by John and developed by Dr. Joel Fuhrman, the nutrient-density scores have dramatically increased sales in the highest-ranking foods. Health-conscious shoppers just needed to know which foods to buy more of, and Whole Foods Market was happy to tell them. Greater sales for Whole Foods Market and better health for the people who shop there: it was a win-win situation.

As you know, nutrient-density scores reflect micronutrient level in relation to calories, which is helpful when shopping for healthy choices. But those digits in no way tie in the environmental expenditure or reflect what resources were required to yield those micronutrients in the food.

> The goal is to get as high a level of health-boosting micronutrients from food, while expending the smallest amount of each natural resource to do so.

So while the British are drawing attention to and quantifying a food's carbon dioxide emissions, and while Whole Foods Market is calculating and displaying its nutrient density, neither system relates one value to the other.

Having had the opportunity to tour and work with both environmental and health experts, I feel as though the members of both groups have excellent perspectives—on their own set of values. Many in the nutrition industry are unfamiliar with the exceptional amount of resources it takes to create sustenance. And the environmental community is unacquainted with the value of nutrient density and therefore with what our resources ought to be providing in exchange for their consumption. And it's certainly not calories.

But in merging the two perspectives, we have the complete picture.

For this reason, I feel it's in our best collective interest to pursue a simple goal: get as high a level of health-boosting micronutrients from food, while expending the smallest amount of each natural resource to do so. That's it.

THE NUTRIENT-TO-RESOURCE RATIO: WHAT IT IS AND WHY IT MATTERS

In an effort to achieve this melding of perspectives, I've put together what I call the "nutrient-to-resource ratio." It takes into consideration both micronutrient gain and natural resource expenditure in the food production process.

When applied, the nutrient-to-resource ratio reveals how misguided our resource expenditure is in our failed attempt to nourish the country.

In Chapter 2, I showed the significant divide between the resources it takes to acquire food from animals and the amount it takes to acquire food from plants. That comparison was based on the conventional calorie-to-calorie or pound-to-pound measure, neither of which addresses the true nutritional makeup of the foods being compared. When we take micronutrients into account as well, that significant divide becomes almost hard to comprehend. Clearly, plant-based whole foods require—by far—the least amount of each resource to produce health-boosting micronutrients.

> I believe it should become standard practice to include a food's nutrient-to-resource ratio on all nutrition labels.

At this time, the information we'd need to calculate the ratio of nutrition from different foods to their draw on land, water, and fossil fuel during their production is not publicly available. I'm working to obtain these numbers so that a comprehensive evaluation system can be developed. Considering the health and environmental benefits of this information, I believe it should become standard practice to include a food's nutrient-to-resource ratio on all nutrition labels. The ratio would give consumers a broader and more comprehensive scope as to what products are, in fact, part of the solution.

However, emission (CO₂e) numbers are available for most foods. With that information, I calculated the nutrient-to-emission ratio for a number of foods, using CO_2e emissions as a measure of exchange for micronutrients.

The first step in calculating the ratio is to establish the amount of CO_2e produced to yield a single calorie of a given food. I then divided the nutrient density of the food by the emissions per calorie, and the result is the nutrient-to-emission ratio. You can find the formula for the calculation of emissions per calorie in "Calculating the Numbers" on pages 310–311, along with the sources of nutrition data I used to determine the nutrient density.

But this would be constantly changing

Here is a sample of nutrient-to-emission ratios I've calculated. Keep in mind that the higher the number, the greater the amount of micronutrients is delivered in relation to the amount of CO_2e released.

Plant-Based Food	Nutrient-to-Emissions Ratio
Almonds	1266
Steamed vegetables (combination of carrots, broccoli, asparagus)	272
Lentils	238

Animal	Nutrient-to-Emissions Ratio
Wild fresh local coho salmon	61
Baked chicken breast	11.6
Poached eggs	6.7
Farmed fresh local salmon	6.6
Domestic cheddar cheese	4
Beef tenderloin steak	1.01

As for the other resources, limited information is available with which to calculate the nutrient-to-resource ratios, so by necessity my assessment is limited too. However, I have worked out the ratios for a few foods. Full calculations for all the numbers in the next sections are given in "Calculating the Numbers" on page 310. There, I've presented the information in snapshot form to give you a quick sense of the draws on each resource that various plant and animal food sources demand. For each resource, I look at foods in pairs to contrast the draw each food makes on the particular resource. Comparing foods illustrates the substantial impact our food choices can have on the environment.

NUTRIENT-TO-ARABLE-LAND RATIO

Wheat, Corn, and Soybeans Versus Beef

As you will see from the calculations in "Calculating the Numbers" on page 310, significantly more arable land is needed to harvest an equivalent amount of micronutrients from beef as from wheat, corn, and soybeans:

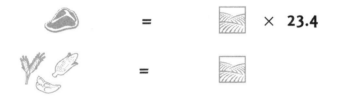

These foods are common feed crops for animals. If we were to use these crops as food for the human population instead, we would gain 23.4 times the amount of micronutrients from the same amount of land.

Hemp Seed Versus Beef

However, if we were to plant hemp as food for humans in place of wheat, corn, and soybeans to feed beef cattle, we would gain 51.9 times the amount of micronutrients on an equal amount of land, compared to what we would obtain from beef.

To explain how I arrive at this figure, by weight, 5.33 times as much hemp seed can be produced as beef raised on the same amount of land (880 pounds of hemp seed per acre[5] compared with 165 pounds of beef[6]). And since beef has a nutrient density of 20 and hemp seed registers at 65 (3.25 times more), for every calorie you get from hemp seed, you'd have to eat 3.25 calories from beef to match the micronutrient level.

Since pound for pound, hemp seed contains about three times more calories than beef, to gain the equivalent in micronutrients from beef as from hemp seed would require 51.9 times more land.

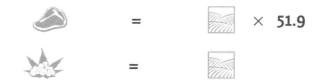

To produce enough beef to match the per-calorie micronutrient level of hemp seed, 51.9 times more arable land would be needed.

Kale Versus Beef

Now, what if instead of growing wheat, corn, or soybeans we grew kale? I realize that comparing kale—among the most efficient and nutrient-dense crops—to beef—one of the worst in both categories—provides something of an extreme case, but the difference *is* impressive. !

By weight, 232 times more kale than cattle can be produced on the same amount of land (38,400 pounds of kale per acre[7] compared with 165 pounds of beef). And since beef has a nutrient density of 20 and kale registers at 1000, which is 50 times greater, for every calorie you get from kale, you'd have to eat 50 from beef to match the micronutrient level.

Since beef has about four times the amount of calories per pound as kale, to gain the equivalent in micronutrients from beef as from kale would require 2900 times more arable land.

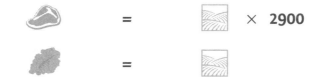

To gain an equal amount of micronutrients from beef as from kale, 2900 times more arable land would be needed,.

NUTRIENT-TO-WATER RATIO

Sweet Potatoes Versus Beef

As mentioned earlier, to produce a pound of beef, a minimum of 2500 gallons of water is required. In contrast, only 60 gallons of water is needed to produce a pound of sweet potatoes, a difference of a little over 41 times. Since beef has a calorie density of 2990 calories per kilogram and sweet potatoes register at 900 calories per kilogram—a difference of 3.3—we can determine that each calorie of beef requires just over 12 times more water to produce than a calorie from sweet potatoes. And since sweet potatoes have a nutrient density of 83, while beef registers at 20—a difference of 4.15—we can determine that a little over 52 times more water is required to gain an equal amount of micronutrients from beef as can be acquired by an equal number of calories from sweet potatoes.

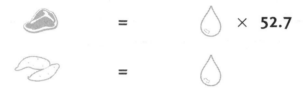

It takes 52.7 times more water to produce an equal amount of micronutrients from beef than from sweet potatoes.

NUTRIENT-TO-FOSSIL-FUEL COMPARISON

Plant Protein Versus Animal Protein

As noted in Chapter 2, the process of acquiring protein from animal sources rather than plant sources uses a great deal more fossil fuel. When we compare micronutrients, that divide becomes even greater. For example, lentils have a nutrient density of 100, whereas the average nutrient density of the animal products listed earlier in this chapter is 25.3. On average, you'd have to eat 3.95 calories from these animal products to obtain the same amount of micronutrients delivered in 1 calorie of lentils. And as mentioned earlier, on average, obtaining protein from animal products requires that

25.4 calories from fossil fuel energy be spent to obtain 1 calorie of protein. And since only 2.2 calories of energy needs to be spent to obtain 1 calorie of protein from lentils, choosing the plant protein equates to an energy savings of 11.5 times (25.4 ÷ 2.2 = 11.5). Multiplying the energy factor by the calorie factor (11.5 × 3.95) tells us that it takes 45.4 times more energy to obtain the same amount of micronutrients from the average animal product as from lentils.

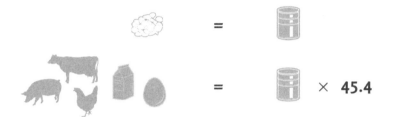

Assuming, for comparison, that the protein amount is equal when factoring in micronutrient levels, 45.4 times more fuel would need to be burned to get an equal amount of micronutrients from animal products as from plants.

Even chicken—the most energy-efficient meat to produce, and a source that is relatively nutrient dense—fares poorly when compared with basic brown rice, which has an average nutrient density, since rice yields more micronutrients while requiring less fossil fuel to produce.

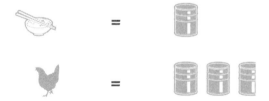

Since rice has a nutrient density of 41 and chicken has a nutrient density of 27, you'd have to eat 1.5 calories of chicken to obtain the same amount of micronutrients as found in 1 calorie of rice. Chicken requires 1.8 times more energy to produce than rice. If you multiply this energy factor (1.8) by the calorie factor (1.5), you'll see that 2.7 times more energy is needed to yield an equal amount of micronutrients.

Since the nutrient density of kale is 10 times that of lentils, 454 times as much fuel would need to be burned to obtain equivalent micronutrients from animal products as from kale.

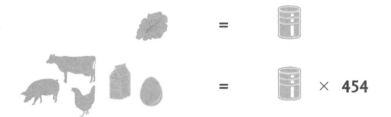

Since the nutrient density of kale is 10 times that of lentils, 454 times more fuel would need to be burned to obtain equivalent micronutrients from animal products as from kale.

Cutting out the intermediary and going directly to the source uses significantly less fossil fuel and is therefore notably more efficient.

NUTRIENT-TO-EMISSION RATIO

In the following examples I use calories as the method of comparison, as opposed to weight or volume. Comparing the amount of emissions required to produce an equal number of calories from a variety of sources gives, I believe, the fairest comparisons. (However, when the ratio is calculated by using weight instead, the discrepancies are even greater. I've listed them below each example.) The complete calculations are in "Calculating the Numbers" on page 310.

Lentils Versus Chicken

Producing meat in the form of a chicken creates the fewest emissions as far as animal agriculture goes. Yet calorie for calorie, chicken emits 5.57 times more CO_2e in its production than lentils. And since lentils are 3.7 times more nutrient dense than chicken (lentils have a nutrient density of 100, and chicken has a nutrient density of 27), 20.6 times more greenhouse gases (5.57×3.7) will be released into the atmosphere to obtain the same amount of micronutrients from chicken as from lentils.

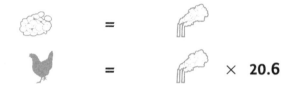

Acquiring an equal amount of micronutrients from chicken
as from lentils would require 20.6 times more CO_2e
to be released into the atmosphere.

When comparing weight instead of calories, pound for pound, the divide would actually be slightly larger, registering at 28.8.

Steamed Vegetables Versus Baked Salmon

Steamed vegetables have a nutrient density average of 304, and salmon has a nutrient density of 39, which means that you'd need to produce 7.8 times more salmon to yield the same nutrient levels of steamed vegetables. Therefore, to obtain the equivalent amount of micronutrients from salmon as from steamed vegetables would mean 41.44 times more greenhouse gases being released into the atmosphere.

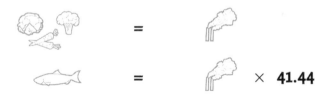

41.44 times more CO_2e would be released into the atmosphere
to gain the equivalent micronutrient content from coho salmon
as from vegetables.

When comparing an equal weight of vegetables to salmon—pound for pound as opposed to calorie to calorie—an even greater divide is revealed. There would be 113.55 times more carbon dioxide released into the atmosphere to gain the equivalent micronutrient content from a pound of coho salmon as from a pound of vegetables.

Nuts Versus Domestic Cheese

Since raw nuts (almonds, cashews, walnuts, pistachios) have an average nutrient density of 36.75, and cheese has a nutrient density of 10, for every calorie obtained from nuts, 3.68 must be obtained from cheese to match the micronutrient content. There would be 2.49 grams of CO_2e released into the atmosphere in the production of 1 calorie from cheese, compared to only 0.03 grams to create a calorie from nuts.

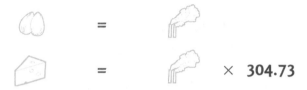

304.73 times more CO_2e would be released into the atmosphere
to gain the equivalent micronutrient content from "American cheese"
as from raw nuts.

Since pound for pound nuts have more calories than cheese, cheese production would emit only 209 times as much carbon dioxide as nut production if the foods were compared on the basis of weight.

Kidney Beans Versus Beef Tenderloin

Just for fun, here's an extreme example: standard factory-farmed beef contrasted with beans.

Kidney beans emit 116 times (CO_2e per calorie of beef tenderloin: 19.72 ÷ 0.17 CO_2e per calorie of kidney beans) less CO_2e than the production of beef tenderloin. Since kidney beans are 5 times more nutrient dense than beef, 580 times (116 × 5) more greenhouse gasses will be released into the atmosphere to gain an equal amount of micronutrients from beef tenderloin compared to kidney beans.

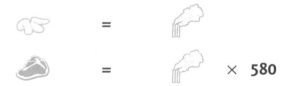

To obtain the same amount of micronutrients from beef as from beans, 580 times
more greenhouse gases would need to be released into the atmosphere.

When comparing equal weight of beans to steak rather than calories, the divide is even greater: 1560 times more carbon dioxide would be released into the atmosphere through the production of beef tenderloin than through the production of beans to produce an equal amount of micronutrients.

THE LOW COST OF HIGH NUTRITION

What about cost? We know that food requiring fewer resources to produce comes at a substantially lower environmental cost. And we know that those same nutrient-rich plant-based whole foods greatly reduce the risk of disease, which will likely translate into a cost savings at both an individual and a societal level. We also know that basing our diet on nutrient-dense whole foods has been shown to reduce sick days per year and enhance mental clarity; hence, a boost in productivity may result, which some may choose to put a dollar value on.

> It's certainly true that more calories and a greater mass of food (or food-like substances) can be had per dollar from highly processed refined sources, but does *nutrition* really cost more?

But what about the upfront monetary cost of healthier food—is it really more expensive? Yes. And no. It's certainly true that more calories and a greater mass of food (or food-like substances) can be had per dollar from highly processed refined sources, but does *nutrition* really cost more? I wondered, since micronutrients are the true measure of a food's worth, what the cheapest way to obtain them might be. Through conventional "standard" foods with lower price stickers? Or by way of plant-based whole foods priced a little higher? Bear in mind that the following examples are based on the retail (government-subsidized) prices for the meat option

The following sections describe what I found out.

Black Beans Versus Eggs

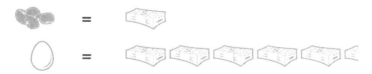

It costs 5.24 times more to gain nutrition from eggs as it does from black beans.

Eggs cost about $3.99 a dozen (about $2.99 per pound), and based on a caloric density of 1430 calories per kilogram, we can determine that each 100 calories costs 46 cents. Since eggs have a nutrient density of 27, their nutrient-to-cost ratio is 58.7 (27 ÷ $0.46). In contrast, black beans cost about $1.59 per pound, and based on a caloric density of 1320 calories per kilogram, each 100 calories from black beans costs 27 cents. Factoring in a nutrient density of 83, black beans have a nutrient-to-cost ratio of 307.41, 5.24 times greater than eggs. Therefore, you would have to eat six eggs, at a cost of $2, to match the micronutrient content you would acquire from 4 ounces of black beans, at an expenditure of 40 cents, a cost difference of over 5 times. ($1.59 [price per pound] ÷ 4 [price per 4 ounces] 0.40 × 5.24 = $2 worth of eggs) (40 cents × 5.24 = $2 [6 eggs])

Lentils Versus Chicken

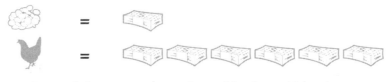

It costs 6 times as much to gain nutrition from chicken breast
as it does from lentils.

Chicken costs about $4.99 per pound, so based on a caloric density of 1650 calories per kilogram, each 100 calories costs 67 cents. Since chicken has a nutrient density of 27, its nutrient-to-cost ratio is 40.30 (27 ÷ $0.67). In contrast, lentils cost about $1.99 per pound, and based on a caloric density of 1060 calories per kilogram, each 100 calories costs 41 cents. Factoring in a nutrient density of 100, lentils have a nutrient-to-cost ratio of 243.9, six times greater than that of chicken. Therefore, you would have to eat 9.5 ounces of chicken, at a cost of $3, to match the micronutrient content you would acquire from 4 ounces of lentils, at a cost of 50 cents, a cost difference of 6 times. ($1.99 [price per pound] ÷ 4 [price per 4 ounces] 0.50 × 6 = $3 worth of chicken) (50 cents × 6 = $3 [9.5 oz of chicken])

Chicken is 2.5 times more expensive by weight: 2.5 ÷ 1.55 = 1.6. Therefore, calorie for calorie, chicken is 1.6 times more expensive than lentils. Lentils are 3.7 times more nutrient dense than chicken: 3.7 × 1.62 = 6.

Therefore, you would have to spend 6 times more to gain equal nutrition from chicken as from lentils.

Flax Versus Coho Salmon

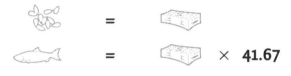

It costs 41.67 times more to gain nutrition from salmon as it does from flax.

Salmon costs about $15.99 per pound, and based on a caloric density of 1900 calories per kilogram, each 100 calories from salmon costs $1.85. Since salmon has a nutrient density of 39, its nutrient-to-cost ratio is 21.08 (39 ÷ $1.85). Flaxseed costs about $1.79 per pound, and based on a caloric density of 5340 calories per kilogram, each 100 calories costs $0.074. Factoring in a nutrient density of 65, flaxseed has a nutrient-to-cost ratio of 878.38, 41.67 times greater than that of salmon. Therefore, you would have to eat 1.17 pounds of salmon, at a cost of $18.78, to match the micronutrient content you would acquire from 4 ounces of flaxseed, at a cost of 45 cents, a cost difference of over 41 times. ($1.79 [price per pound] ÷ 4 [price per 4 ounces] 0.45 × 41.67 = $18.75 worth of salmon) (45 cents × 41.67 = $18.75 [1.17 pounds of salmon])

WHY DOES A HAMBURGER COST LESS THAN AN APPLE?

Have you ever wondered how it is that meat and other highly processed food—all of which consumes an inordinate amount of land, water, and oil to produce—costs relatively little in dollars? How is it that a hamburger at a fast food restaurant can cost under $2 when a locally grown organic apple that uses a fraction of the energy to produce it costs the same or more? The short answer: government subsidies. In the United States, these happen through legislation known as the Farm Bill—the government's chief food policy tool. While it was introduced with the best of intentions, the Farm Bill has veered off course and no longer benefits the people as a whole. And certainly not the planet.

The original aims of the bill were achieving food security and helping struggling farmers make enough money to stay in business. However, the subsidies were misdirected. They began to flow mostly to the meat and dairy industry. Even with strong sales, the production cost of meat and dairy was simply too high (because of its substantial resource cost, in turn because of inefficiency) to enable farmers to make a profit. Had the government not stepped in and bailed out this exceptionally inefficient industry with monetary subsidies, the cost of meat and dairy would be prohibitive to almost everyone. Instead, subsidies turned these products into cheap commodities, causing consumption to skyrocket—and with it, pollution and disease. To rub salt in the wound, we're paying for it. Government money comes from the taxpayers. So, even those of us who don't support these inefficient industries by patronizing them prop them up by way of the current tax system. And now, to reopen the wound and dump more salt in, we also highly subsidize our reactive medical systems, which pours money into treating symptoms caused by poor-quality diets made possible, and encouraged, by subsidies. It truly is a vicious cycle.

> "Pay now for healthier food, or pay later to treat the symptoms of disease as a result of poor nutrition."

It's estimated that the health costs from poor diet are $250 billion per year in the United States alone, and the U.S. National Institutes of Health (NIH) has predicted that obesity will lower Americans' life expectancy by up to five years over the next few decades.

In 2006, I had an opportunity to speak to the U.S. Congress about exactly this issue: the Farm Bill. I've learned that when speaking to such governmental groups, it's important to focus on one thing: money. So I did. My suggestions were along the line of preventative medicine. I presented information suggesting that if subsidies were to be lifted, people simply would not be able to afford resource-gobbling food; they would have to eat simple plant-based foods. The most nutrient-dense food would then be the cheapest. Its lower cost would, of course, give people an economic incentive to eat better food. And, as a direct result, the disease risk factor of poor nutrition would be much reduced and the overworked health-care system would be much relieved of its strain. While nothing of significance developed as a result of my presentation, the nodding heads in the audience indicated

Don't expect the gov't to make any dramatic change.

that the simple logic of "Pay now for healthier food, or pay later to treat the symptoms of disease as a result of poor nutrition" seemed to strike a chord.

Considering the immense resource draw of meat production, it seems reasonable to say that if meat were sold at a fair market value, consumption of it would plunge. People simply wouldn't be able to afford it. Estimates on the fair market price for a typical fast-food burger, costed without subsidies, range from $35 all the way up to $200. The $35 calculation is based on the fossil fuel cost to produce it, while the $200 figure includes the land and water costs. In addition, the $200 burger price factors in the delivery of the food to the feedlots, and the cleanup of the water systems polluted by the cattle's manure. But, as it stands, with taxpayer-funded subsidies, this same hamburger at a fast-food restaurant will go for about $2. Sometimes as low as $1—if you select the "value menu" and agree to buy a carton of fries and a soft drink.

THE GREAT ENVIRONMENTAL DIVIDE: MEAL PLAN COMPARISONS

Following are three sample one-day meal plans to further illustrate the environmental impacts of our food choices. In each I've calculated and compared the amount of CO_2-equivalent emissions each meal is responsible for releasing during its production.

The first meal plan reflects the Standard American Diet, subsistence in the form of processed food-like substances, which relies heavily on red meat and dairy, with very little food in its natural state.

Second, I look at the "healthy" American diet. The go-to diet for many Americans once they've begun to experience health decline from years of eating the Standard American Diet, the "healthy" American diet is only marginally less processed and far from a long-term health solution. And, as I found, the amounts of CO_2-equivalent emissions created by its production are enough to be of major environmental concern.

The third meal plan is devised following the nutritional philosophy of this book: it uses plant-based whole foods with a high nutrient-to-resource ratio.

The numbers next to each meal are the grams of CO_2-equivalent emissions (here, CO_2e for short) released into the atmosphere in the production of the food composing each meal.

STANDARD AMERICAN DIET

Breakfast: Omelet with meat and cheese; cereal and milk; 12 oz coffee with cream and sugar. CO_2e: 3101 g

Lunch: Cheeseburger and fries; 12 oz soft drink. CO_2e: 3116 g

Dinner: Beef stir-fry; 12 oz beer; milk chocolate bar for dessert. CO_2e: 3387 g

TOTAL CO_2e: 9604 g

"HEALTHY" AMERICAN DIET

Breakfast: Buttermilk pancakes; scrambled eggs with cheese; latte. CO_2e: 2661 g

Lunch: Baked farmed salmon; 5 oz wine. CO_2e: 1396 g

Dinner: Chicken Caesar salad; baked potato with sour cream; 12 oz water. CO_2e: 1317 g

TOTAL CO_2e: 5374 g

WHOLE FOODS TO THRIVE SUGGESTION

Breakfast: Nutrient-dense plant-based smoothie (containing hemp protein, pea protein, rice protein, and flaxseeds) blended with banana and blueberries. CO_2e: 130 g

Snack: Seasonal fruit and nuts. CO_2e: 104 g

Lunch: Vegetable stir-fry and lentils. CO_2e: 361 g

Snack: Oven-roasted potatoes. CO_2e: 84 g

Dinner: Beans and rice with grilled vegetables and green salad. CO_2e: 308 g

Snack: Raw vegetables and hummus. CO_2e: 212 g

TOTAL CO_2e: 1199 g

So what do these numbers actually mean? That's what I wondered. To make them relatable, I've compared the CO_2-equivalent emissions released in food production with the CO_2 emissions created from driving. What I found was striking.

The chart on the next page shows the grams of CO_2-equivalent emissions that each diet would produce over various periods: a day, a week, a month, a year. I then compare these CO_2 levels with what's produced by different driving distances.

For a midsize car that averages between 26 and 28 miles per gallon, about half a pound (227 g) of carbon dioxide is released into the atmosphere to travel one mile.[8] Knowing that, we can directly compare driving with eating and its impact on the environment.

However, because the numbers for the consumption of arable land, water, and fossil fuel are not yet available for all food products, in the examples I use only CO_2-equivalent emissions to compare food's impact on the environment. Needless to say, the environmental toll is far greater when all factors are considered.

CO₂-equivalent emissions Diet by time period compared to driving distance		
Emissions from diet		Emissions from driving
STANDARD AMERICAN DIET		
Day: 9604 grams	=	42.4 miles
Week: 67,240 grams	=	296 miles
Month: 291,961 grams	=	1,289 miles
Year: 3,505,460 grams	=	15,476 miles
"HEALTHY" AMERICAN DIET		
Day: 5374 grams	=	23.7 miles
Week: 37,618 grams	=	166 miles
Month: 163,397 grams	=	720 miles
Year: 1,961,510 grams	=	8,650 miles
WHOLE FOODS TO THRIVE SUGGESTION		
Day: 1199 grams	=	5.28 miles
Week: 8393 grams	=	37 miles
Month: 36,469 grams	=	160.65 miles
Year: 437,635 grams	=	1928 miles

Sources of data: www.falconsolution.com/co2-emission/
227 g (1/2 lb) CO_2 to travel 1 mile in midsize car
Driving distances are for a midsize car that averages between 28 and 30 miles per gallon.

The contrasts among the diets are dramatic, to say the least.

But headlining just about every "what you can do to save the planet" list is the suggestion that we abstain from driving, or at least greatly reduce the amount we do. "Ride your bike, take transit, or—if you must—carpool." To many, driving has become a sign of environmental disregard. And while I agree that using alternative means of transportation and depending less on the automobile makes sense, are cars really deserving of so much attention?

Clearly, with automobile transportation we have a hands-on relationship. We regularly need to fill our vehicles with gasoline. This gives us an idea as to how much fuel we directly consume. Besides, filling up costs money, which for the average person reinforces the value of fossil fuel. That's good. Most of us appreciate the value of gas because of its high and ever-increasing cost and have a sense of the environmental damage its combustion is causing. We see the emissions spewing from tailpipes as we drive around. And sitting in rush-hour traffic, if we roll down the window, we experience directly how CO_2 emissions are adversely affecting air quality. Over cities such as Los Angeles, we can see a thick layer of smog engulfing the buildings as a direct result of tailpipe exhaust. And as such, we have a close, tangible, and therefore relatable relationship with our vehicle and its fossil fuel–burning, emission-creating ways.

> Making wise food choices can have a more significant impact on environmental preservation than eliminating driving altogether.

In contrast, we don't see the fuel needed in the production of food, and the emissions it releases are not apparent to the average person. But it's real nonetheless. And, as I mentioned earlier when I cited the 2006 U.N. report, the level of these emissions is considerably higher than that released by the automobile.

Toward the bottom of "planet-saving" suggestions, eating locally may sometimes be mentioned. And *maybe* switching to more plant-based options will round out the list. Maybe. But is the weighting of these suggestions reflective of the biggest environmental offenders?

We all have to eat, and making wise food choices can have a more significant impact on environmental preservation than eliminating driving altogether.

Difference in emissions created (equivalent to miles driven) from eating a Standard American Diet compared with Whole Foods to Thrive suggestions	
Day	37.12 miles
Week	259.84 miles
Month	1129 miles
Year	13,549 miles

In just one day, anyone who switched from the Standard American Diet to Whole Foods to Thrive would conserve the equivalent in emissions of the grams released in driving a little over 37 miles. Just one week of eating the Thrive way rather than the Standard diet would conserve as much CO_2e as is released driving 250 miles, the equivalent of traveling by car from Boston to New York City.

Spanning a year, the CO_2e savings would equal the grams emitted in driving from Los Angeles to New York City four-and-a-half times.

Since the average distance driven by each American is 12,500 miles per year,[9] switching from a Standard American Diet to a Whole Foods to Thrive way of eating would prevent more CO_2-equivalent emissions from entering the atmosphere than would abstaining from driving altogether.

Therefore, an average American can do more to mitigate climate change by changing what he or she eats than by completely cutting out driving.

And as for the "healthy" American diet?

Aware of the immense amount of methane and nitrous oxide that raising ruminants, such as cows and sheep, produces, some looking to reduce their carbon footprint are turning to meat from other animals. As you can see from the "healthy" American meal plan, it contains no meat from ruminants, yet its production still releases 338 percent more CO_2e than the suggested plant-based Whole Foods to Thrive meal plan. The environmental culprits in the "healthy" American meal plan? Fish, chicken, and dairy. While emitting less total CO_2e than the Standard American Diet, the "healthy" diet's switch to "white" meat is clearly not the best solution for environmental sustainability. And as mentioned in Chapter 1, such a diet's micronutrient level is considerably lower than we can obtain directly from plants.

4 EIGHT KEY COMPONENTS OF GOOD NUTRITION

While micronutrient density is the best gauge of a food's true nutritional worth, the eight components described in this chapter point to the specifics of what comprise healthy food. Six of the eight are directly related to nutrient density; the other two (whether a food contains essential fats or is a raw food) are not but do contribute to what constitutes a healthy choice.

As you can see, I've assigned an icon to represent each element of nutrition. In the next chapter, "Nutrient-Dense Whole Foods to Thrive," you can look for these icons as a quick key to identify the foods that are the top sources of each element.

ALKALINE-FORMING FOODS

The measure of acidity or alkalinity is called pH, and maintaining a balanced pH is an important part of reaching and sustaining peak health. The body can become more acidic through diet and, to a lesser degree, through stress. Since minerals are exceptionally alkaline-forming, the pH of any food is largely dependent on mineral content. Returning to the subject of soil quality, even greens—which are highly alkaline-forming due to their chlorophyll content—will not be as alkaline-forming if they are grown in mineral-depleted soil.

Alkaline-forming foods help to balance the body's pH. An acidic environment adversely affects health at the cellular level; people with low body pH are prone to fatigue and disease. And because acidity is a stressor, it raises cortisol levels, which results in impaired sleep quality.

To help your muscles recover and to lower your cortisol levels, consume highly alkalizing foods, such as those rich in chlorophyll, soon after exercise. Chlorophyll is the green pigment that gives leaves and green vegetables their color.

BEST SOURCES
- All green vegetables
- Seaweed
- Algae

BENEFITS
- Improves bone strength
- Reduces inflammation
- Improves muscle efficiency
- Reduces risk of disease

 ## ANTIOXIDANTS

As mentioned in Chapter 2—in the first section, "Arable Land"—plants are only capable of producing antioxidants if they have drawn an adequate amount of minerals from the soil. For plants to develop their full antioxidant potential, they must be grown in mineral-rich soil.

> Antioxidant compounds found in fruits and vegetables cancel out the effects of the cell-damaging free radicals by slowing or preventing the oxidative process.

When our body's activity level rises, we use extra oxygen, which causes cellular oxidation. Oxidation can create free radicals, which reduce cell lifespan and cause premature cell degeneration. Damage done by free radicals has been linked to cancer and other serious diseases and to premature skin aging. Free radicals occur naturally in the body, with small amounts being produced daily, but stress can increase their presence. A reduction of stress through better nutrition combats the oxidative process and therefore free radical production. Antioxidants in foods also help to rid the body of free radicals by escorting them out of the body.

Because of the increased oxygen consumption associated with regular strenuous physical activity, it creates an abundance of free radicals. We therefore need to combat this negative side effect of exercise. Antioxidant compounds found in fruits and vegetables—vitamin C, vitamin E, selenium, and the carotenoids (compounds that give vegetables their orange color)—cancel out the effects of the cell-damaging free radicals by slowing or preventing the oxidative process. I noticed a clear improvement in how fast I recovered between workouts once I regularly began eating antioxidant-rich foods.

BEST SOURCES

- Organic berries
- Organic dark-colored fruit in general
- Organic colorful vegetables
- Green tea

BENEFITS

- Protects cellular health
- Speeds physical recovery
- Reduces risk of disease
- Improves skin's appearance and elasticity

CALCIUM

Since calcium is a mineral, the amount present in food has been declining over the years. Again, food quality is dependent on soil quality.

For most people, building, strengthening, and repairing bone is calcium's major role. Active people, however, have another important job for the mineral: muscle contraction and rhythmic heartbeat coordination. About 95 percent of the body's calcium is stored in the skeleton, but it's the remaining share that is the first to decline. Calcium in the bloodstream is lost in sweat and muscle contractions, so active people need more dietary calcium. Another micronutrient, vitamin D, maximizes calcium absorption. Vitamin D comes from the sun, so regular exposure to daylight will help your body absorb calcium and therefore help with bone maintenance.

Over the course of about the last 15 years, North Americans have been losing bone density and developing osteoporosis at a younger age than ever before in history. Initially, this loss was thought to be due to inadequate dietary calcium. Advertisements in magazines and on TV tried to convince people over the age of 40 to take calcium supplements. Unfortunately, the body doesn't properly absorb the inorganic forms of calcium found in supplements, so we'd need to consume a very large amount for supplementary calcium to have even a small impact on bone health. The net-gain principle suggests that the consumption of inorganic calcium is a poor use of energy. In fact, it's not uncommon for people who take calcium supplements to notice an energy dip within an hour or so after taking them.

Plants take inorganic calcium from the soil and convert it into an organic form of calcium that the human body can efficiently and completely make use of. Consuming an adequate supply of organic calcium from such sources as leafy green vegetables ensures that our bones stay strong and that muscle contractions remain smooth and efficient.

We must also make sure we don't remove the calcium that already exists in our bodies, so it's important to avoid acid-forming foods, which deplete our stores of calcium and so weaken the bones.

BEST USABLE PLANT SOURCES
- Dark leafy greens, such as spinach, kale, collard greens
- Unhulled sesame seeds

BENEFITS
- Improves muscle function and efficiency
- Increases bone strength
- Reduces the risk of osteoporosis

ELECTROLYTES
Electrolytes are electricity-conducting salts drawn from the soil. Calcium, chloride, magnesium, potassium, and sodium are the chief electrolyte minerals. Electrolytes in body fluid and blood regulate or affect the flow of nutrients into cells and of waste products out of cells, and are

essential for the regulation of muscle contractions, heartbeats, fluid levels, and general nerve function. When too few of these minerals are ingested, we may suffer muscle cramps and heart palpitations, light-headedness and trouble concentrating. In severe cases, lack of electrolytes leads to loss of equilibrium, confusion, and inability to reason.

You may have noticed salt-like crystals forming on your face when you perspire heavily. Those are electrolytes—what's left when the water component of sweat has evaporated—and they have to be replenished through food and drink. But not just any drink. When we consume too much fluid that does not contain electrolytes, it can flush out the remaining electrolytes from our body, referred to as water intoxication. While it isn't common among the general population, people who perform strenuous physical activity, especially in a warm environment, are susceptible.

Most commercial sports drinks contain unnecessary refined sugar and artificial flavor and color. Soon after my own experience with water intoxication, I developed my own formula for a natural, healthy, electrolyte-packed drink, my Lemon-Lime Sports Drink (the recipe is on page 130).

BEST SOURCES
- Coconut water
- Molasses and molasses sugar
- Seaweed (dulse and kelp in particular)

SECONDARY SOURCES
- Bananas
- Tomatoes
- Celery

BENEFITS
- Helps maintain hydration
- Improves the fluidity of muscle contractions
- Increases the heart's efficiency, lowers heart rate, improves endurance
- Boosts mental clarity

ESSENTIAL FATS

Essential fatty acids (EFAs) are an important dietary component of overall health. The word *essential* in the name means the body cannot produce these fatty acids—they must be ingested. There are two families of EFAs, omega-3 and omega-6.

EFAs support the function of the cardiovascular, immune, and nervous systems. Studies suggest that including omega-3, in particular, in the diet can benefit those who suffer from a wide range of ailments, including high blood pressure, high cholesterol, heart disease, diabetes, rheumatoid arthritis, osteoporosis, depression, bipolar disorder, schizophrenia, attention deficit disorder, skin disorders, inflammatory bowel disease, asthma, colon cancer, breast cancer, and prostate cancer.[1] These studies also suggest that an adequate supply of omega-3 may help reduce the risk of developing these ailments in the first place.

> EFAs play an integral role in the repair and regeneration of cells and therefore in keeping the body biologically young.

Responsible in part for the cells' ability to receive nutrition and eliminate waste, EFAs play an integral role in the repair and regeneration of cells and therefore in keeping the body biologically young. A balance of omega-3 and omega-6 EFAs will keep skin looking and feeling supple. EFAs also help fight infection and reduce inflammation. In addition, EFAs are linked to healthy and efficient brain development in children.

From an active person's perspective, when combined with proper endurance training, a diet with an adequate supply of EFAs can help improve endurance. Our bodies can store only a small amount of muscle carbohydrate. Once the body has burned all of its carbohydrate stores, it has to be refueled—as often as every 30 minutes during a long race or workout. However, once the body has adapted to a period of long, slow training (as I describe in my book *Thrive Fitness*), it becomes more efficient at burning body fat as fuel and thus is able to preserve its carbohydrate stores. This shift in metabolism is simply a trait of improved fitness, which therefore enables the body to burn less fuel to travel the same distance. This fuel shift means that refueling doesn't have to take place as often and endurance will be significantly improved. The fuel shift is facilitated by dietary EFAs, which need to be properly balanced between omega-6 and omega-3 to be effective. The ideal ratio is said to be 4:1. For every four parts omega-6 that's in your diet, you'll want to have one part omega-3. Fortunately, a plant-based whole food diet naturally provides that ratio.

BEST SOURCES

These all contain a balance of omega-3 and omega-6.

- Sacha inchi
- Chia
- Flaxseed
- Hemp

BENEFITS

- Improves endurance
- Increases the body's ability to burn body fat as fuel
- Improves the ability to stay well hydrated
- Improves joint function

IRON

Drawn into plant plasma from the soil, iron helps maintain blood cell health so that the heart can deliver oxygen-rich blood to the hardworking extremities—maximizing efficacy and therefore athletic performance. Iron also builds blood proteins essential for food digestion, metabolism, and circulation.

Iron is lost in sweat and is consumed during muscle contraction. The pounding impact of our feet on the ground during running can cause red blood cells to break down and thus lower their iron levels. People with low iron are at risk for anemia. Dietary iron helps counteract these problems.

About eight years ago, I went through a stage of reduced energy and poorer performance. I had a blood test to find out what was wrong. It showed that my iron level was low—not so low that I couldn't train at all, but certainly low enough to hinder my progress. I had borderline anemia. Because my active lifestyle consumed a lot of iron and because I did not eat animal products, which are higher in iron than plant-based foods, my doctor suggested I begin taking iron in tablet form. I knew a few people who had experienced stomach problems and even constipation when they began their iron supplementation program, so I wanted to see whether I could get all the iron I needed just from food. I found there are many good plant-based sources of iron. For me, a combination of about ¼ cup raw pumpkin seeds and a green salad daily did the trick. Within a few months my iron levels were back to optimal and have remained there ever since.

BEST PLANT-BASED SOURCES

- Pumpkin seeds
- Leafy greens (especially kale)
- Vega Complete Whole Food Health Optimizer (contains 100 percent of the recommended daily allowance)

BENEFITS

- Improves blood's oxygen-carrying ability
- Increases physical stamina
- Boosts energy

PHYTONUTRIENTS

Since phytonutrients are a specific form of antioxidants, they, along with other antioxidants, can only be produced if their host plant is grown in mineral-rich soil.

Phytonutrients are plant compounds that offer health benefits independent of their nutritional value. They are not essential for life, but they can help improve vitality and quality of life.

For example, a phytonutrient found in tomatoes improves blood vessel elasticity and thereby enhances blood flow through the heart. Tomatoes can thus lower the risk of developing cardiovascular disease and enhance athletic performance. The heavy processing of fruit and vegetables reduces the amount and effectiveness of phytonutrients, so these foods are best eaten raw. Every type of fruit and vegetable has at least a few phyto-nutrients, so simply eating many servings on a daily basis will boost health and performance.

BEST SOURCES
- Colorful and green vegetables

BENEFITS
- Improves heart health
- Reduces the risk of cardiovascular disease
- Improves blood vessel elasticity, thereby improving circulation

 RAW FOOD

As I noted earlier, eating a large percentage of raw food makes sense on several levels. High-temperature cooking and processing of food destroys enzymes and nutrients needed for efficient digestion. Before the body can make use of cooked food, it must produce enzymes to aid in the digestion process. That takes work, which of course is an energy draw and therefore creates a nominal amount of stress. In addition, food containing both sugar and fat cooked at a high temperature can provoke an immune response that causes inflammation. However, minerals are not damaged by heat, so cooking food will not lower mineral content. Vegetables that contain a high amount of starch, such as potatoes and sweet potatoes, are best eaten cooked.

BEST SOURCES
- Fruit
- Nuts
- Seeds
- Most vegetables

BENEFITS
- Improves digestibility of most (non-starchy) foods
- Maintains higher vitamin content in most foods
- Allows for higher net gain and therefore more energy

As you'll see, these beneficial traits are a large component of the foods that are the base ingredients for the recipes in Chapter 6.

5 NUTRIENT-DENSE WHOLE FOODS TO THRIVE

The whole foods I'll tell you about in this chapter are among the prime ingredients in the recipes to follow in Chapter 6. And, as you might expect, they are among the most nutrient-dense foods there are while requiring less of each natural resource to produce than more traditional foods. As you can see, I've used the icons representing the eight key components of nutrition to indicate when a particularly high amount of a certain component is present in the food. These icons serve as a quick visual guide as to which foods are richest in these elements. These foods are essential components of daily meals in the Whole Foods to Thrive plan so I call them "Pantry Essentials"; you should make sure you have them on hand at all times.

WHOLE FOODS TO THRIVE PANTRY ESSENTIALS

Green Vegetables

Alkaline-Forming   Antioxidants   Calcium   Electrolytes   Essential Fats   Iron   Phytonutrients   Raw

Because of their chlorophyll content, green vegetables are an excellent way to help alkalize the body, which, as I mentioned before, reduces inflammation and helps maintain bone health.

Chlorophyll also cleanses and oxygenates the blood, making it a true performance enhancer. More available oxygen in the blood translates into better endurance and an overall reduction in fatigue. In their raw state, chlorophyll-containing plants also possess an abundance of live enzymes that promote the quick rejuvenation of our cells. The consumption of green foods after exercise has been shown to help speed cellular regeneration. The consumption of chlorophyll-rich leafy green vegetables combined with moderate exercise is the best way to create a biologically younger body. Ounce for ounce, dark greens are also an excellent source of iron and calcium.

> The consumption of chlorophyll-rich leafy green vegetables combined with moderate exercise is the best way to create a biologically younger body.

You may not crave a plate full of fibrous, leafy green vegetables immediately after exercise, and they'd take up room in your stomach needed for other post-recovery nutrition. An easy way to ingest greens immediately after exercise is to mix a greens powder, such as chlorella or spirulina, into a fruit-based post-exercise recovery drink (the "Drinks" recipes start on page 128). Later in the day, a big salad is an ideal way to load up on more leafy greens.

All leafy greens are nutrient-dense and an excellent conduit for minerals in the soil; here are some of the more readily available ones:

- Beet greens
- Butter lettuce
- Collards
- Dandelion greens
- Dinosaur kale
- Mustard greens
- Red leaf lettuce
- Romaine lettuce
- Spinach
- Swiss chard

Fibrous Vegetables

Also mineral-rich, these vegetables are high in both soluble and insoluble fiber:

- Asparagus
- Beets
- Bok choy
- Broccoli
- Carrots
- Celery
- Cucumbers
- Daikon
- Green beans
- Green peas
- Green onions
- Sugar snap peas
- Watercress
- Zucchini

Starchy Vegetables

SQUASH

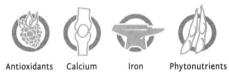

Antioxidants   Calcium   Iron   Phytonutrients

There are several types of squash, all with distinctly different flavors and textures; butternut, spaghetti, acorn, carnival, banana, zucchini, delicata, and kabocha are among the most popular and therefore the most common.

The most nutrient-dense form of starch-based food, squash is an excellent addition to the diet. Especially of value for those who aspire to pack on muscle, squash—combined with the correct workout—will contribute to the process of muscle building.

Many varieties of squash are grown in North America and can be found at most farmers' markets, especially in the autumn.

Other starchy vegetables include

- New potatoes
- Parsnips
- Pumpkin
- Sweet potatoes
- Yams

Sea Vegetables

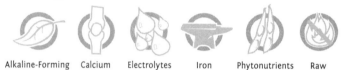

Alkaline-Forming   Calcium   Electrolytes   Iron   Phytonutrients   Raw

Sea vegetables, often referred to as seaweed and less commonly as wild ocean plants, have been a staple of many coastal civilizations for thousands of years. Most notably, Asian cultures have long since embraced sea vegetables as an important part of their diet.

Sea vegetables are among the most nutritionally dense foods. Containing about 10 times the calcium of cow's milk and several times more iron than red meat, sea vegetables are easily digestible, chlorophyll rich, and alkaline forming. Packed with minerals, sea vegetables are the richest source of naturally occurring electrolytes known.

Dulse, nori, and kelp are the most popular sea vegetables in North America. Available in dried and ready-to-use form in most health food stores, their addition to many recipes is easy. Dulse provides the perfect mineral balance in a natural form and so is a superior source of the minerals and trace elements we need daily for optimal health.

Other, less common, sea vegetables are agar, arame, kombu, and wakame.

Pseudograins

Commonly referred to as grains but technically seeds, pseudograins are naturally gluten free and contain more protein (20 percent to 25 percent by volume) and are higher in micronutrient density than grains. You can use pseudograins in most recipes calling for rice.

BUCKWHEAT

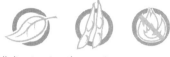

Alkaline-Forming Phytonutrients   Raw

Buckwheat is not actually wheat; it is a seed in the rhubarb family.
Containing eight essential amino acids, including quite high amounts of the
often-elusive tryptophan, buckwheat is a good source of protein. Tryptophan
is a precursor to the neurotransmitter serotonin; having an adequate amount
of tryptophan in the diet can be important to help enhance mood and
mental clarity. Buckwheat is also high in vitamins E and B, calcium, and
especially manganese.

Since buckwheat is gluten free, it is considerably more alkaline
forming than gluten-containing grains. It is also a slow-release carbohydrate. Combined with a simple carbohydrate, buckwheat becomes one of
the best endurance fuels available. Sprouted buckwheat digests and burns
even more effectively because the sprouting process converts the complex
carbohydrate into sugar, which the body can burn more efficiently than
starch. But since the protein, fat, and fiber remain, this sugar will not cause
an insulin spike and subsequent crash. Raw buckwheat can also be substituted for seeds in recipes to reduce fat content.

QUINOA

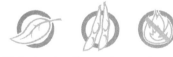

Alkaline-Forming Phytonutrients   Raw

With a light, fluffy texture and mild earthy taste, quinoa balances the
texture of other, heavier grains when combined with them.

Nutritionally similar to amaranth, quinoa consists of about 20 percent
protein; it is high in lysine and is a good source of iron and potassium. High
levels of B vitamins, in part responsible for the conversion of carbohydrate
into energy, are also found in quinoa.

The preparation of quinoa is particularly important since it is naturally
coated in a bitter resin called saponin. Thought to have evolved naturally to
deter birds and insects from eating the seed, saponin must be removed by

thorough rinsing to make quinoa palatable. Most of the saponin will have been removed before the quinoa is shipped to the store, but there will likely be a powdery residue.

Cook quinoa like rice, at a 1:2 quinoa-to-water ratio, for about 20 minutes. Quinoa can also be sprouted (Google "sprouting quinoa" for instructions).

WILD RICE

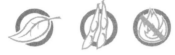

Alkaline-Forming Phytonutrients Raw

Wild rice is an aquatic grass seed rather than a true rice. High in B vitamins and the amino acid lysine, wild rice is much more nutritious than traditional grains. Native to the northern regions of the Canadian Prairie provinces, wild rice is seldom treated with pesticides since it thrives without them. (It is also grown as a domesticated crop in Minnesota and California.) Wild rice has a distinct, full-bodied flavor and a slightly chewy texture that complement many meals.

Cook like rice, at a 1:2 wild rice-to-water ratio, for about 30 minutes. It can also be sprouted (Google "sprouting wild rice" for instructions).

Seeds

FLAXSEED

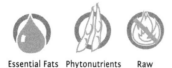

Essential Fats Phytonutrients Raw

Grown mostly in the Canadian prairies, the seed of the blue-flowering flax plant is prized for its lignans and high omega-3 fatty acid content. The regular inclusion of lignans in the diet has been shown to reduce the risk of cancer. Flaxseed is also rich in fiber. However, it is its omega-3 essential fat content that makes flaxseed most valuable to athletes. As I noted earlier, aside from its ability to help reduce inflammation caused by movement, omega-3 plays an integral role in the metabolism of fat. A diet with a daily dose of 1 tablespoon of whole flaxseed will allow the body to more efficiently burn body fat as fuel. This is obviously a benefit to anyone wanting to shed body fat, but it is of major importance to athletes, who need to spare the energy stored in the muscles. As the body becomes proficient at burning fat as fuel (through training and proper diet), endurance significantly improves.

Whole flaxseed is high in potassium, an electrolyte responsible in part for smooth muscle contractions. Potassium is lost in sweat, so it must be replaced regularly to keep the body's levels adequately stocked. Potassium also helps to maintain fluid balance, assisting with the hydration process. Flaxseed is a whole food and a complete protein, and it retains its enzymes, allowing it to be absorbed and utilized by the body with ease, improving immune function.

HEMP SEEDS

Alkaline-Forming   Essential Fats   Phytonutrients   Raw

Hemp is available in three basic forms: seed, powder, and oil. Hemp seeds come straight from the plant and are rich in both omega-3 and omega-6 essential fatty acids. When pressed, the seed becomes hemp powder and oil. The powder, sometimes referred to as flour, is then milled finer to remove some of the starch. The result is hemp protein.

The protein present in hemp is complete, containing all 10 essential amino acids, which boost the immune system and hasten recovery. Hemp foods also have natural anti-inflammatory properties, key factors for speeding the repair of soft tissue damage caused by physical activity. Raw hemp products maintain their naturally high level of vitamins, minerals, high-quality balanced fats, antioxidants, fiber, and the very alkaline chlorophyll. Edestin, an amino acid present only in hemp, is considered an integral part of DNA. It makes hemp the closest plant source to our own human amino acid profile.

When it comes to protein, quality, not quantity, is paramount. I find hemp protein the easiest protein to digest. Since it is raw, its naturally occurring digestive enzymes remain intact. That and its relatively high pH allow it to be easily used by the body. As a result, the digestive strain placed on the body to absorb and utilize protein is reduced, making it a high-net-gain food. Top-quality, complete protein, such as hemp, is instrumental not only in muscle tissue regeneration but also in fat metabolism. Protein ingestion instigates the release of a hormone that enables the body to more easily utilize its fat reserves, thereby improving endurance and facilitating body fat loss.

PUMPKIN SEEDS

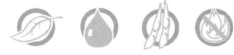

Alkaline-Forming   Essential Fats   Phytonutrients   Raw

Pumpkin seeds are rich in iron, a nutrient some people have trouble getting enough of, especially if they don't eat red meat. Anemia, a shortage of red blood cells in the body, is commonly caused by low dietary iron or by strenuous exercise. Iron is lost as a result of compression hemolysis (crushed blood cells due to intense muscle contractions). The more active the person, the more dietary iron she needs. Constant impact activity, such as running, reduces iron levels more dramatically than other types of exercise because of the more strenuous hemolysis. With each foot strike, a small amount of blood is released from the damaged capillaries. In time, this will lead to anemia if the runner doesn't pay close attention to her diet. Iron is also lost through sweat.

SESAME SEEDS

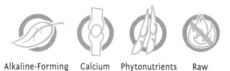

Alkaline-Forming   Calcium   Phytonutrients   Raw

Sesame seeds are an excellent, easily absorbable source of calcium. Calcium is in part responsible for muscle contractions—of particular concern to athletes, who will need to ensure that they maintain correct levels of calcium in the body. Calcium plays another important role in the formation and maintenance of bones and teeth. Athletes and people living in a warm climate will need extra amounts of dietary calcium since it is excreted in sweat.

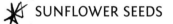

I use a coffee grinder to grind sesame seeds into a flour, then store it in the refrigerator, for up to three months. I sprinkle the flour on salads, cereal, pasta, and soups. Some of the recipes in Chapter 6 call for sesame seed flour, to increase calcium content. When baking, it's possible to substitute sesame seed flour for up to one-quarter of the amount of regular, glutinous flour called for in the recipe. If the recipe calls for non-glutinous flour, the whole amount can be replaced with sesame seed flour. However, since sesame seed flour is slightly more bitter than most flours, you may want to experiment, gradually increasing the amount each time.

SUNFLOWER SEEDS

Phytonutrients   Raw

Made up of about 22 percent protein, sunflower seeds offer a good amount of dietary substance. Rich in trace minerals and several vitamins important for good health, sunflower seeds are a food worthy of regular consumption. Sunflower seeds are quite high in vitamin E and are antioxidant rich.

Legumes

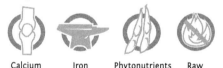

Calcium   Iron   Phytonutrients   Raw

Legumes are plants that have pods containing small seeds. Lentils, peas, and beans are all in the legume family. Lentils and split peas are among the most commonly used legumes in this book's recipes for the simple reason that they don't need to be soaked before cooking.

Legumes in general have an excellent nutritional profile. High in protein, fiber, and many vitamins and minerals, a variety of legumes are part of my regular diet. Peas, and in particular yellow peas, have an exceptional amino acid profile. Also rich in B vitamins (in part responsible for converting food into energy) and potassium (an electrolyte needed for smooth muscle contractions), yellow peas are an excellent addition to an active person's diet. Because of peas' superior amino acid profile, manufacturers are now producing pea protein concentrates and isolates. This high-quality vegetarian protein is a good option for people with soy allergies.

Although some people avoid legumes because of their gas-producing reputation, legumes are no more a culprit than many other foods as long as they are prepared properly. After you have soaked beans and shelled peas in preparation for cooking, be sure to rinse them in fresh water. Rinse them again in fresh water after cooking. The water they soak and cook in will absorb some of the indigestible sugars that cause gas; rinsing it off will help improve their digestibility and minimize their gas production. Another way to improve the legumes' digestibility is to add seaweed to the pot when cooking them, to release the gas. A short strip of seaweed is enough for a medium-sized pot. As with all fiber-rich foods, legumes should be introduced slowly into the diet to allow time for the digestive system to adapt. Gradually increasing the amount of legumes you eat each day will ensure a smooth transition to a healthier diet.

Raw legumes are ideal for sprouting. Sprouting improves both legumes' nutritional value and their digestibility—enough so that they may be eaten raw. As well, sprouting allows the digestive enzymes to remain intact, eliminating gas production altogether.

These are the legumes I suggest for their nutritional value and taste:

- Adzuki beans
- Black beans
- Chickpeas*
- Fava beans
- Kidney beans
- Lentils
- Navy beans
- Pinto beans
- Yellow and green split peas

Oils

Oils come in a wide assortment, each with a distinct taste and unique nutritional value. The key to keeping the flavors in your meals ever changing and your diet's nutrient value diverse is using various oils.

In the right amount, high-quality, cold-pressed, unrefined oils are among the healthiest of substances. My favorites are hemp, pumpkin, flaxseed, and, for cooking, coconut. Most oils contain the same nutrients as the plant seed they are from, just highly concentrated.

Not all oils are equal. Low-quality manufactured oil is one of the most damaging foods that can be consumed, eclipsing even refined carbohydrate. Many cheaper store-bought baked or fried products, such as muffins, chips, and cakes, contain trans fat, a near-poisonous substance unusable by the body. Trans fat, also known as trans-fatty acid, is added to many mass-produced commercial products to extend their shelf life, improve moisture content, and enhance flavor. ***BAD.***

As for the oils used in the Whole Foods recipes, it's helpful to know which can be heated safely and which are best consumed raw. I never fry with hemp, flaxseed, or pumpkin seed oil because of their low burning point—the temperature point at which oil becomes molecularly damaged. Exceeding the burning point can convert healthy oils into trans-fatty acids. When baking with ingredients that contain fatty acids, such as flaxseed and other milled seeds, it is important that the temperature not exceed 350 degrees Fahrenheit. I rarely bake anything at temperatures above 300 degrees Fahrenheit, to ensure the fatty acids retain their nutritional value. For stir-frying, when the temperature is likely to exceed 350 degrees Fahrenheit, I use only coconut oil.

COCONUT OIL

Raw

Coconut oil is produced by pressing the meat of the coconut to remove the fiber. This is the only fat I use for frying. Sometimes called coconut butter since it's solid at a temperature below about 80 degrees Fahrenheit, coconut oil can be heated to a high temperature without converting to a trans fat. Surprisingly, coconut oil does not have a strong coconut taste, and it has almost no smell. When used in cooking, any remaining hint of the coconut taste leaves, making it a versatile oil.

Coconut oil is rich in medium-chain triglycerides, or MCTs. MCTs are unique in that they are a form of saturated fat yet have several health benefits. The body utilizes them differently from fat that does not contain MCTs. Their digestion is near-effortless and, unlike fat that does not contain MCTs (which gets stored in the cells), MCTs are utilized in the liver. Within moments of MCTs being consumed, they are converted by the liver to energy. It's for these properties that I include coconut oil in my energy gel recipes, beginning on page 275. They provide easily digestible energy, ideal during activity such as cycling or hiking.

EXTRA-VIRGIN OLIVE OIL

Raw

"Extra-virgin" means that the oil is from the first pressing of the olive. The subsequent pressing is referred to as virgin, the one following that produces regular olive oil. With a light taste and color, extra-virgin olive oil is a healthy addition to sauces, dips, and dressings. Although extra-virgin olive oil is a healthy oil, it delivers only minimal amounts of omega-3.

FLAXSEED OIL

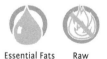

Essential Fats   Raw

As you would expect, flaxseed oil is obtained by pressing flaxseed. Milder in taste than hemp and pumpkin seed oils, flaxseed oil contains the highest amount of omega-3 in comparison to omega-6, at a 5:1 ratio.

Ideal ratio of Omega 6 to Omega 3 is 4:1.
(See page 99)

HEMP OIL

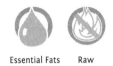

Essential Fats   Raw

Obtained by pressing hemp seed, hemp oil is one of the healthiest oils available. Dark green with a smooth creamy texture and mild, nutty flavor, hemp oil is an excellent base for salad dressings. Hemp oil is unique in that it has the ideal ratio of omega-6 and omega-3 fatty acids.

PUMPKIN SEED OIL

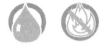

Essential Fats   Raw

Pumpkin seed oil is a deep green color with a hint of dark red. With a distinct, robust flavor, pumpkin seed oil is packed with essential fatty acids and has been linked to improved prostate health.

Nuts

ALMONDS

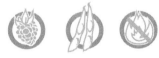

Antioxidants   Phytonutrients   Raw

The almond is one of the most popular nuts in North America. Almonds are resistant to mold without being roasted, making them a perfect nut to soak and eat raw. Particularly high in vitamin B2, fiber, and antioxidants, almonds have one of the highest nutrient levels of all nuts. That, combined with their high level of digestibility, especially when soaked, makes them a worthy addition to your diet. Although almonds don't need to be soaked, soaking makes them more nutritious—in this pre-sprouting state, their vitamin levels increase and the enzyme inhibitors are removed, making them even more efficiently digested.

MACADAMIA NUTS

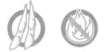

Phytonutrients   Raw

Macadamia nuts contain omega-7 and omega-9 fatty acids. While these are nonessential fatty acids, meaning the body produces them, their inclusion in the diet has been linked to positive health benefits. Blending soaked macadamia nuts results in a creamy spread that makes for a healthy alternative to butter or margarine. Although soaked macadamia nuts are recommended for any of my recipes calling for macadamia nuts, they don't need to be soaked if you're short of time or unprepared.

WALNUTS

Electrolytes Phytonutrients   Raw

Walnuts are rich in B vitamins and possess a unique amino acid profile. Also rich in potassium and magnesium, walnuts can help maintain adequate electrolyte levels in the body, prolonging hydration. As with almonds and macadamia nuts, soaking improves their nutrition and digestibility. Walnuts complement many meals and snacks.

OTHER NUTS

The nuts listed below all offer high levels of nutrition in a compact form. These nuts can be substituted in recipes for the more common nuts, such as almonds and macadamia. Because of their diversity, incorporating them into your diet will ensure a greater variety of taste and nutrition. However, these nuts may not be readily available in grocery stores.

- Brazil nuts
- Cashews
- Filberts
- Hazelnuts
- Pecans
- Pine nuts
- Pistachios

Hazelnut trees grow wild in Europe and Asia. A staple in early humans' diet, hazelnuts have been eaten for thousands of years. Filberts are a variety of hazelnut that are cultivated and are often produced larger than wild hazelnuts to increase crop yield. Wild hazelnuts and filberts are nutritionally similar; both are excellent sources of the minerals manganese, selenium, and zinc.

Grains

As for true grains—as opposed to pseudograins—brown (or whole-grain) rice is my first choice. It's gluten free and offers considerably more micronutrients than other grains.

BROWN RICE

Phytonutrients

A staple of many countries, rice is one of the most consumed foods in the world by volume. Since brown rice has been unaltered over the years, the possibility of it causing an allergic reaction is low. Brown rice has a mild, nutty flavor.

The processing of brown rice is far less extensive than that of white rice, making it nutritionally superior to its white counterpart. Since only its outermost layer, the hull, is removed, brown rice retains its nutritional value. Brown rice is very high in manganese and contains large amounts of selenium and magnesium. It is a good source of B vitamins as well.

Purple sticky rice, or Thai black rice, is a nice alternative to standard brown rice. It can be substituted for brown rice at a 1:1 ratio.

Cook at rice-to-water ratio of 1:2. Put rice and water in a pot. Cover and bring to a boil. Once it's boiling, reduce heat to a simmer; simmer for 45 minutes. Remove from the stove and stir. Let cool.

Fruit

Pretty much all fruit is good. As mentioned in Chapter 1, fruit as a source of carbohydrate is considerably easier to digest than refined flour products and offers a significantly higher micronutrient density, hence rendering it a high-net-gain food. Therefore, making fruit the prime carbohydrate source instead of grain products will translate into greater usable energy.

Dates

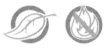

Alkaline-Forming   Raw

Dates are nearly pure glucose, which, in its natural form, is a valuable type of sugar for people who are active. Glucose is rapidly converted to glycogen in the liver. Maintaining an adequate glycogen supply in both the muscles and the liver is imperative for sustained energy. For that reason, dates are best consumed shortly before, during, or immediately following exercise. Chlorophyll-rich foods also convert to glycogen, but not as quickly as glucose, therefore making the easily digestible, alkaline-forming date the ideal snack to fuel activity.

I use dates as the base ingredient for my whole food energy bar recipes starting on page 271.

Ginger

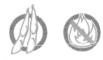

Phytonutrients   Raw

Fresh ginger is a worthy addition to any diet. Ginger can help the digestion process and ease an upset stomach. I use it in many recipes. Ginger has anti-inflammatory properties and so aids in the recovery of soft-tissue injuries and helps promote quicker healing of strains. I load up on ginger as my mileage increases to ensure inflammation is kept under control.

Green Tea

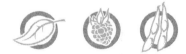

Alkaline-Forming   Antioxidants   Phytonutrients

While green, or incompletely fermented, tea leaves do contain a form of caffeine, it differs significantly from the form found in coffee beans. Theophylline causes a slow, steady release of energy over the course of several hours. Therefore, it does not cause caffeine jitters and places less stress on the adrenal glands. Green tea is also rich in chlorophyll and antioxidants.

However, since green tea is classified as a stimulant, it is something that I suggest drinking only before physical exercise. Green tea can help improve the level of intensity a person can reach during a workout or on race day. This leads to better, faster results. Theophylline has also been shown to help improve focus and concentration and to calm nerves. Before a big race, being able to relax and focus are valuable traits.

NEXT-LEVEL FOODS

These foods are sometimes harder to source; not all grocery stores will carry them, but most health food stores will. While these foods typically score among the top in terms of nutrient-to-resource ratio, they are not essential for healthy living. They will, however, provide a boost of nutrition in a concentrated form.

Kombucha

Alkaline-Forming   Antioxidants   Electrolytes   Phytonutrients   Raw

A popular health elixir in Asia, kombucha is a fermented tea, rich in organic acids, active enzymes, amino acids, and antioxidants. Its fermentation results in "good" bacteria content that helps improve the body's digestive strength, enabling it to metabolize and utilize nutrition more quickly. Additionally, kombucha acts as a natural muscle relaxant, helping muscles move with greater fluidity and ease, resulting in less energy expenditure and, ultimately, enhanced endurance. This is why I include a small amount of kombucha in my pre-workout drink. Also a liver detoxifier, kombucha helps speed cellular recovery. You'll find a basic kombucha recipe on page 133.

Where may I find this. *I still need to try the kit Holly bought me!*

Sacha Inchi

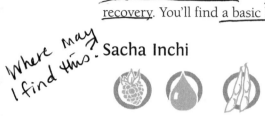

Antioxidants   Essential Fats   Phytonutrients

With a green star-shaped fruit that yields a highly nutritious seed, the sacha inchi plant is native to the Peruvian Amazon. Also know as the "Incan peanut," the seed has several health properties, including easily digestible protein. High levels of the amino acid tryptophan are also present, making the seed a natural mood enhancer that lowers the risk of brain chemistry imbalances and depression. An exceptionally good source of omega-3 and omega-6 essential fatty acids, sacha inchi is among the most concentrated sources of omega-3 in the plant kingdom, coming in at 48 percent by volume. Also high in vitamin A and E, sacha inchi is rich in antioxidants. (For more information on sacha inchi, please visit saviseed.com.)

Palm Nectar

Phytonutrients

Also known as coconut palm sugar, palm nectar is a low-glycemic form of natural sugar. Made from the sap of the date or coconut palm tree much as maple syrup is tapped from the maple tree, it is an ideal source of sustainable energy. It can be used as a low-glycemic sweetener, or as a premium, easily digestible fuel source that's ideal before a workout. Combining it with a high-glycemic sugar, such as that from dates or sprouted rice, I use palm nectar to balance the glycemic profile and slow the rate at which the sugar enters the blood stream.

Açaí Berries

Antioxidants   Electrolytes   Essential Fats   Phytonutrients   Raw

Açaí berries are the small, purple fruit of palm trees that grow in marshy areas in Central and South America, where it has been eaten by native people for centuries.

The berries are exceptionally rich in antioxidants and contain essential fatty acids and amino acids. Because they are also easy to digest, açaí are a high-net-gain food that can speed recovery after exercise.

In North America, açaí can be bought in most health food stores either frozen whole or freeze-dried in powdered form. The frozen berries are handy for making a smoothie. And you can mix the powder into recipes such as energy bars as an easy way to boost nutritional content.

Chlorella

Alkaline-Forming   Antioxidants   Essential Fats   Phytonutrients   Raw

Nutritionally speaking, chlorella—a fresh-water green algae—is a true superfood, comprising 67 percent protein; essential fatty acids; and a plethora of vitamins, minerals, and enzymes. Chlorella contains vitamin B12, which is difficult for vegetarians and vegans to find in forms other than laboratory-created tablets. Chlorella also possesses all 10 of the essential amino acids—the ones that must be obtained through diet for peak health. These amino acids, in conjunction with naturally occurring enzymes, are the most easily absorbed and utilized form of protein available. Many other complete proteins are much more energy-intensive to digest; by comparison, chlorella is a particularly high-net-gain food. Spirulina is also an excellent form of fresh water algae. While its protein content and B vitamin levels are lower than that of chlorella, it is still highly alkaline forming.

Coconut Water

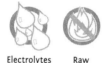

Electrolytes   Raw

Coconut water is the nearly translucent fluid inside the coconut (not to be confused with coconut milk, which is a combination of coconut water blended with coconut meat). It has a light, sweet flavor. It is fat-free and contains high levels of simple carbohydrates, making it an ideal fluid to boost muscle glycogen without causing the stomach to become bogged down with digestive duties.

Packed with electrolytes, coconut water is the original sports drink. It has been used for decades to properly hydrate people who sweat profusely in tropical regions.

Maca

Phytonutrients

Maca, a root vegetable with medicinal qualities, is native to the high Andes of Bolivia and Peru. Known as an adaptogen, maca curtails the effects of stress by aiding the regeneration of the adrenal glands, making it an ideal food for the modern world. It helps lower cortisol levels, which will improve sleep quality. Of course, better-quality sleep directly translates into more waking energy. And maca increases energy by means of nourishment, not stimulation. I have found that I am better able to adapt to physical stress when I add maca to my diet.

Maca is a rich source of steroid-like compounds found in both plants and animals that promote quick regeneration of fatigued muscle tissue. During the off-season, I make a concerted effort to build strength and muscle mass in the gym. I've recently experienced exceptional strength gains by adding maca to my recovery drink. I can lift more weight than in previous years and I recover faster. It has enabled me to perform more high-quality workouts, thereby advancing my progress.

Published human clinical studies of maca used the gelatinized form of the vegetable. Gelatinization removes the hard-to-digest starchy component of the maca root. The result is an easily digestible, quickly assimilated, and more concentrated form of maca. Gelatinized maca has a pleasant, nutty taste and dissolves more easily than regular maca. When selecting maca, be sure to choose the gelatinized form for best results.

Chia

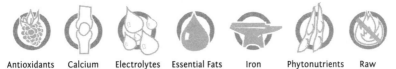

Antioxidants Calcium Electrolytes Essential Fats Iron Phytonutrients Raw

Chia seeds are small and round and look like white poppy seeds. Grown in the Amazon basin in Peru, chia laps up the nutrients in the rich, fertile soil and passes them on to the consumer. With a unique crunchy texture, chia is gaining in popularity in North America.

Particularly high in magnesium, potassium, calcium, and iron, chia can effectively replenish minerals used in muscle contractions and lost in sweat. Chia is truly one of the top foods for active people. And because it is high in both soluble and insoluble fiber, which helps to sustain energy and maintain fullness, chia is a true high-net-gain food. Packed with antioxidants and containing about 20 percent high-quality protein, chia is an ideal food to help speed recovery after exercise.

Aztec warriors were rumored to eat chia before going into battle to give them a nutritional boost and thereby improve their endurance. They were also said to have carried it with them when they ran long distances to be used as their body's primary fuel source. Since chia is nutritionally well rounded and complete, this may well have been the case. It is ideal to help maintain energy level during a workout, and the seeds are remarkably easy to digest.

Yerba Maté

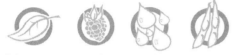

Alkaline-Forming Antioxidants Electrolytes Phytonutrients

Yerba maté is a species of holly native to subtropical South America. The leaves are rich in chlorophyll, antioxidants, and numerous trace minerals, and help aid digestion. However, since yerba maté does contain a form of caffeine, I suggest drinking it in a similar fashion to green tea, before exercise or when you really need extra short-term energy.* Yerba maté is one of the healthiest forms of stimulation, yet any kind of stimulation will take its toll on the adrenal glands eventually.

However, after drinking yerba maté, it's important to make sure the adrenals are well nourished to help speed recovery. I include maca in my post-workout drink for this reason.

When sourcing yerba maté, it's of course best to avoid products from plantation-style farms that have cleared old-growth forest. Be sure to choose a brand that is wild harvest or has been grown with the jungle, not instead of the jungle. By making the harvesting of wild yerba maté economically viable for the producers, you will help prevent clearance of old-growth rain forest for the farming of animals. Before yerba maté rose to popularity outside of South America, it was common for large plots of land to be clear-cut for cattle-grazing land. While this is still a problem, in those areas with an abundance of yerba maté growing within the jungle, the yerba maté can be harvested without any alteration to the forest canopy; therefore, using the jungle to grow yerba maté enhances the "value" of the natural foliage so that in many cases there is more incentive to preserve it rather than to convert it to cattle pasture.

Part of a food forest ☺

Stevia

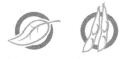

Alkaline-Forming Phytonutrients

Stevia is a herb native to Paraguay. The intense sweetness of its leaf
is stevia's most celebrated feature. About 30 times as sweet as sugar,
dried stevia leaf contains no carbohydrates and so does not affect the body's
insulin levels. Stevia has been shown to help equalize blood sugar levels
raised by other sugars and starch consumed at the same time. Stevia, as you
might expect, is quickly gaining popularity as a natural sugar substitute
among those in pursuit of a leaner body. Improved digestion is another of
stevia's benefits. An excellent alternative to manufactured artificial sweeteners, stevia leaf is a whole food, just dried and ground into powder. When
choosing stevia, be sure you read the ingredients; it's commonly combined
with maltodextrin and other fillers. Selecting a stevia brand with stevia as
the sole ingredient is ideal. I add it to many of my foods. Its ability to help
regulate blood sugar levels is important for sustained energy. I even add
stevia to my sports drink to improve its effectiveness.

6

WHOLE FOODS RECIPES

drinks

Sunflower Seed Hemp Milk (and Chocolate Variation)

I usually make a week's supply of Sunflower Seed Hemp Milk at a time, which for me is about 8 cups. Hemp milk is a good substitute for cow's milk on cereal. For a tasty change, try using the chocolate version on your morning cereal. Hemp milk also adds a subtle creaminess and flavor to smoothies.

Time: 2 minutes • <u>Makes about 3 cups</u>

2 ½ cups water
½ cup hemp seeds
½ cup sunflower seeds

3 large pitted dates (fresh, or dried
    dates soaked overnight)
1 tbsp roasted carob powder or cocoa
    powder (for chocolate variation)

- In a blender, combine all ingredients and blend until smooth. To make into chocolate milk, you may add 1 tbsp of either roasted carob powder or cocoa powder before blending. Be aware that cocoa, unlike carob, does contain a bit of caffeine.
- Keep refrigerated, for up to 2 weeks.

Sacha Inchi Milk (and Chocolate Variation)

Soaking sacha inchi seeds doesn't enhance their nutritional value, but it does allow them to be blended into a smooth milk.

Time: 2 minutes • Makes about 3 cups

2 ½ cups water
1 ½ cups soaked sacha inchi seeds
3 large pitted dates (fresh, or dried dates soaked overnight)
2 tbsp roasted carob powder or cocoa powder (for chocolate variation)

- In a blender, combine all ingredients and blend until smooth. To make into chocolate milk, you may add 2 tbsp of either roasted carob powder or cocoa powder before blending. Be aware that cocoa, unlike carob, contains a bit of caffeine.

Ginger Pear Smoothie with Sunflower Seed Hemp Milk

The riper the pear, the sweeter the smoothie. If you'd like it even sweeter, add one or two fresh or soaked dried dates. Since ginger is a natural anti-inflammatory, this is an ideal choice for a post-workout snack.

Time: 2 minutes • Makes about 3 cups (2 servings)

1 banana
½ pear, cored
1 cup water
1 cup Sunflower Hemp Seed Milk (see p. 128)
1 tbsp ground flaxseed
1 tbsp hemp protein powder
1 tbsp peeled, grated ginger

- In a blender, combine all ingredients and blend until smooth.

Chocolate Almond Smoothie with Sacha Inchi Milk

Rich in protein and omega-3, this smoothie will keep you going for hours with sustainable, non-stimulating energy.

Time: 5 minutes • Makes about 3 ½ cups (2 large servings)

1 banana
2 fresh or presoaked dried dates
1 cup water
1 cup Sacha Inchi Milk (or chocolate variation) (see p. 128)
¼ cup almonds (or 2 tbsp raw almond butter)
1 tbsp ground flaxseed
1 tbsp hemp protein powder
1 tbsp roasted carob powder

- In a blender, combine all ingredients and blend until smooth.

Brendan's Original Lemon-Lime Sports Drink

Dates are high in glucose, which will enter the blood stream almost instantly. The sugar in the coconut water will enter the blood stream more slowly, spreading out the energy over a longer period.

Fresh dates are ideal. You can also soak dried dates for four hours beforehand to rehydrate.

Time: 5 minutes active • Makes 2 cups (1 large serving)

1 cup coconut water

1 cup water

2 dates (pitted fresh or presoaked dried)

Juice from ½ lemon

Juice from ¼ lime

Sea salt to taste

- In a blender, combine all ingredients and blend. If you prefer your drink smooth, strain out any pulp left from the lemon and lime.

The Brazier

THRIVE JUICE BAR, WATERLOO, ONTARIO

Jonnie Karan, co-founder of Thrive Juice Bar, named this one after me since he figured I'd like it. He was right. It's certainly one of my favorites.

Time: Under 5 minutes prep • Makes 2 cups

1 tsp raw cocoa nibs

1 tbsp organic cocoa powder

6–7 raw cashews

2 tsp blue agave nectar

¼ tsp vanilla extract

1 scoop or 1 ¾ ounces organic dairy-free
   vanilla gelato

1 tbsp almond butter

⅓ ripe banana

⅓ cup rice milk

½ cup coconut water

2 or 3 ice cubes

- In a blender, combine all ingredients, including ice, and blend until smooth.
- It's best served immediately but can be kept up to 2 days in the fridge.

Thai Avocado Smoothie

THRIVE JUICE BAR, WATERLOO, ONTARIO

A unique-flavored and filling smoothie.

Time: Under 5 minutes • Makes 2 cups

½ ripe avocado
3 tsp dark raw agave
1 tsp vanilla extract
½ tsp chopped lemongrass

½ cup coconut water
⅓ cup rice milk
2 or 3 ice cubes

- In a blender, combine all ingredients, including ice, and blend until smooth.
- It's best served immediately but can be kept up to 2 days in the fridge.

Coconut Thai Lime Leaf Smoothie

THRIVE JUICE BAR, WATERLOO, ONTARIO

Lime leaf adds extra chlorophyll and a whole bunch of extra flavor in this exotic-tasting smoothie

Time: Under 5 minutes • Makes 2 cups

2 small scoops or ½ cup non-dairy
   coconut gelato
2 tsp blue agave
½ tsp chopped lemongrass
3 medium Thai lime leaves (available,
   usually frozen, in Asian markets)

Zest of half a lime
⅓ cup rice milk
½ cup coconut water
2 or 3 ice cubes

- In a blender, combine all ingredients, including ice, and blend until smooth.
- It's best served immediately but can be kept up to 2 days in the fridge.

Coconut, Mango, Yellow Curry Smoothie

THRIVE JUICE BAR, WATERLOO, ONTARIO

Straight-up delicious with anti-inflammation properties as a bonus from the curry.

Time: Under 5 minutes • Makes 2 cups

½ cup frozen mango
1 fresh orange, juiced
½ tsp lime, juiced
⅛ tsp yellow curry powder
2 tsp blue agave

¼ cup rice milk
2 ounces organic pure mango juice
⅓ cup coconut water
2 or 3 ice cubes

- In a blender, combine all ingredients, including ice, and blend until smooth.
- It's best served immediately but can be kept up to 2 days in the fridge.

La Belle Verte (The Beautiful Green One) Smoothie

CRUDESSENCE, MONTREAL, QUEBEC

Sweet, chlorophyll-rich goodness.

Time: Under 5 minutes • Makes 2 cups

¾ banana, frozen (or fresh banana
    + 2–3 ice cubes)
4 chunks pineapple
2 large leaves fresh kale
¼ cup parsley, chopped (firmly packed)

1 or 2 dates
2 tbsp shelled hemp seeds
1 pinch sea salt
1 ½ cups water

- Place all ingredients in a blender and add water to 16-ounce level. Blend until texture is like a smoothie, without lumps.
- It's best served immediately but can be kept up to 2 days in the fridge.

Kombucha Mojito

Delicious, nutritious, and refreshing. Can be served solo, or with a meal to aid in digestion.

Time: 5 minutes • Makes 2 servings

½ cup chopped mint
3 tbsp fresh squeezed lime juice
2 tbsp orange juice
3 tbsp palm sugar

½ tsp lime zest
Ice
2 cups kombucha
Mint leaves, for garnish

- Muddle the mint, lime juice, orange juice, palm sugar, and lime zest together to release the flavor of the mint leaves.
- Strain and pour into 2 glasses filled with ice. Top each glass with kombucha, stir, and top with a fresh mint leaf for garnish.

Green Mango Dessert Smoothie

Is it a smoothie or is it a dessert? The Vega Sport Performance Protein Powder with its 20 grams of protein, high-quality ingredients, and smooth texture pretty much rocks in this recipe, but another vanilla hemp or rice protein will work too. You can increase the protein powder to two servings and add a little extra water for a less dessert-like, more traditional smoothie.

Time: 5 minutes • Makes 2 servings

2 heaping cups frozen mango chunks
½ cup hemp milk
½ cup water
1 scoop vanilla-flavored Vega Sport
    Performance Protein Powder

Touch of white stevia, to taste
    (optional)
2 tbsp shredded coconut (optional)

- In a blender, combine mangoes, hemp milk, water, and protein powder and blend until completely smooth.
- If desired, boost sweetness with a touch of stevia, to taste, and blend again. Serve in a bowl and top with shredded coconut.

Pomegranate Smoothie

This is a simple, refreshing smoothie.

Time: 5 minutes • Makes about 3 ½ cups (2 large servings)

1 banana
1 date
2 cups cold water (or 1 ½ cups water plus 1 cup ice)
1 cup pomegranate seeds (the amount from 1 pomegranate)
1 tbsp ground flaxseed
1 tbsp hemp protein
1 tbsp hemp oil
½ tsp cayenne pepper

- In a blender, combine all ingredients, and blend until smooth.
- Can be kept up to 3 days in the fridge.

Tropical Pineapple Papaya Smoothie

A good smoothie when you are on the go or feeling fatigued. A great tasting energy booster.

Time: 5 minutes • Makes about 3 ½ cups (2 large servings)

1 banana
2 fresh or soaked dried dates
2 cups cold water (or 1 ½ cups water plus 1 cup ice)
½ medium papaya
½ cup pineapple
1 tbsp ground flaxseed
1 tbsp hemp protein
tbsp coconut oil

- In a blender, combine all ingredients, and blend until smooth.
- Can be kept up to 3 days in the fridge.

Chocolate Goodness Smoothie

A full-flavor, nutrient-dense, chlorophyll-rich super smoothie that's filling enough to take the place of a meal.

Time: 5 minutes • Makes 1–2 servings

1 banana
1 cup frozen blueberries
1 cup unsweetened hemp milk
1 scoop Chocolate Vega Complete Whole Food Health Optimizer
1 tsp wheatgrass powder
2 tbsp raw cocoa powder
1 tsp mesquite powder
Stevia powder, to taste (substitute a touch of palm sugar
    or maple syrup if desired)
2–3 cups water
Handful of ice

- In a blender, combine all ingredients, including ice, and blend until smooth.

Toasted Chia Ginger Pear Cereal

With significant amounts of omega-3 and ginger, this cereal is considerably less acid-forming than standard ones. To make it even more nutritious, top with an energy bar cut into small pieces (recipes starting p. 266).

Time: 10 minutes prep; 1 hour to bake • Makes 4 cups (about 5 servings)

½ pear, diced
1 cup oats (or cooked or sprouted quinoa, to make cereal gluten free)
½ cup diced almonds
½ cup chia seeds
½ cup hemp protein
½ cup unhulled sesame seeds
½ cup sunflower seeds
¼ tsp ground stevia leaf
¼ tsp sea salt
¼ cup hemp oil
¼ cup molasses
2 tbsp apple juice
1 tbsp grated ginger root
Coconut oil

- Preheat oven to 250°F.
- In a large bowl, combine pear, oats, almonds, chia seeds, hemp protein, sesame seeds, sunflower seeds, stevia, and sea salt. In a small bowl, blend together hemp oil, molasses, apple juice, and ginger root. Add wet ingredients to dry ingredients, mixing well.
- Spread on a bake tray lightly oiled with coconut oil. Bake for 1 hour. Let cool, then break into pieces.
- Keeps refrigerated for up to 2 weeks.
- Eat with Sunflower Seed Hemp Milk (see p. 128) or Sacha Inchi Milk (see p. 128).

Sacha Inchi Baked Apple Cinnamon Cereal

With high-quality protein and omega-3 and omega-6 essential fatty acids, this cereal is filling. A great way to make it even more nutritious is to top it with an energy bar cut into small pieces (recipes start on p. 272).

Time: 10 minutes prep; 1 hour to bake • Makes 4 cups (about 5 servings)

½ apple, diced
1 cup oats (or cooked or sprouted quinoa, to make cereal gluten free)
½ cup diced sacha inchi seeds
½ cup ground flaxseed
½ cup hemp protein
½ cup unhulled sesame seeds
½ cup sunflower seeds
1 ½ tsp cinnamon
¼ tsp nutmeg
¼ tsp ground stevia leaf
¼ tsp sea salt
¼ cup hemp oil
¼ cup molasses
2 tbsp apple juice
Coconut oil

- Preheat oven to 250°F.
- In a large bowl, combine apple, oats, sacha inchi, flaxseed, hemp protein, sesame seeds, sunflower seeds, cinnamon, nutmeg, stevia, and sea salt. In a small bowl, blend together hemp oil, molasses, and apple juice. Add wet ingredients to dry ingredients, mixing well.
- Spread on a baking tray lightly oiled with coconut oil. Bake for 1 hour.
- Let cool, then break into pieces.
- Keeps refrigerated for up to 2 weeks.
- Eat with Sunflower Seed Hemp Milk (see p. 128) or Sacha Inchi Milk (see p. 128).

Breakfast Blueberry Chia Pudding

Since chia rapidly absorbs fluid and takes on gelatinous properties when soaked, it makes an ideal nutrient-dense pudding base.

Time: 5 minutes active; 20 minutes total • Makes about 1 ½ cups (1 serving)

2 tbsp chia
¾ cup water
⅓ cup cashews
2–3 fresh pitted dates, or dried
    pitted dates soaked in water
    overnight to rehydrate

Pinch of cinnamon
Pinch of sea salt
Fresh or frozen blueberries

• Soak chia in water for 15 minutes. In a blender, combine with the rest of the ingredients, except the blueberries, and blend until smooth. Transfer to serving bowl and top with blueberries.

Chocolate Raspberry Chia Pudding

A delicious and filling breakfast.

Time: 5 minutes active; about 35 minutes total
Makes about 2 cups (1 large serving)

4 tbsp chia seeds
½ cup water
1 cup Sunflower Seed Hemp Milk (see p. 128)
1 tbsp cocoa
1 tbsp maple syrup
Raspberries, fresh or frozen

• Soak chia in water for 15 minutes. In small bowl, mix chia, water, and Sunflower Seed Hemp Milk together. Stir for 1–2 minutes or till consistent texture is reached. Add cocoa and maple syrup. Stir and then let sit for 10–15 minutes. As an option, it can be heated on the stovetop for about 2 minutes on low. Stir again, top with raspberries, and serve.

New Potato Pancakes

These whole food carbohydrate-rich pancakes will supply hours of sustainable energy, ideal a few hours before a long hike or bike ride. Use as many kinds of potatoes as possible, such as blue/purple potatoes, fingerlings, round white potatoes, and red potatoes.

Time: 15 minutes • Makes 8 medium-sized pancakes

1 pound mixed, unpeeled, new potatoes
3 tbsp ground flaxseed
2 tbsp brown rice flour
¼ tsp sea salt
1 carrot, shredded
About 1 tbsp coconut oil

- Using a hand grater or food processor, shred the potatoes (if using a food processor, pulse a couple of times using the S-blade after shredding, to make sure the potato shreds are not too long).
- In a small bowl, blend the flaxseed, flour, and salt.
- In a large bowl, toss the shredded potatoes and carrots together, then add in the dry mixture and combine. Use your hands to form 8 palm-size flat patties, about ½-inch thick. Set the patties aside on paper towels to absorb any excess moisture.
- In a large frying pan, heat about a tablespoon of coconut oil over medium high heat. When the oil is hot, add 4 patties. After a few minutes, when the patties are golden brown on the underside, flip them over and cook until the second side is crispy. When patties are cooked, transfer them back to paper towels to remove any excess oil until you are ready to serve them.
- Add a bit of new oil to the pan, and repeat with the remaining patties.

Buckwheat Banana Pancakes

Lightly flavored with cinnamon and nutmeg, these pancakes taste just like traditional pancakes.

Time: 15 minutes • Makes 2 large servings

1 cup buckwheat flour
¼ cup ground flaxseed
¼ cup hemp flour
2 tsp baking powder
1 tsp cinnamon
½ tsp nutmeg
1 banana
2 cups water
½ cup barley flakes (or buckwheat, sprouted or cooked)

- In a bowl, mix buckwheat flour, flaxseed, hemp flour, baking powder, cinnamon, and nutmeg.
- In a food processor, process the banana and water while slowing adding the dry ingredients until mixture is smooth. Stir in the barley flakes with a spoon or spatula.
- Lightly oil a pan with coconut oil and heat over medium heat. Pour in pancake batter to desired pancake size and cook for about 5 minutes or until bubbles begin to appear. Flip and allow to cook for another 5 minutes.

Blueberry Pancakes

Packed with taste and nutrition, these pancakes are a breakfast favorite.

Time: 15 minutes   •   Makes 2 large servings

2 fresh or soaked dried dates
1 cup blueberries
1 cup hemp milk
¾ cup water
½ cup buckwheat flour
½ cup sprouted or cooked quinoa
1 tsp baking powder
1 tsp baking soda
Sea salt to taste

- In a food processor, process all ingredients until smooth
- Lightly oil a pan with coconut oil and heat over medium heat. Pour in pancake batter to desired pancake size and cook for about 5 minutes or until bubbles begin to appear. Flip and allow to cook for another 5 minutes.

HEMP MILK

3 ½ cups water
1 cup hemp seeds
2 tbsp agave nectar

- In a blender, combine all ingredients. Keep refrigerated for up to 2 weeks. Makes about 4 cups.

Wild Rice Yam Pancakes

This is a heartier mixture than traditional pancakes, one that will give you a sense of fullness for several hours.

Time: 15 minutes • Makes 2 large servings

2 cups water
1 cup cooked or sprouted quinoa
1 cup mashed cooked yam
½ cup sprouted or cooked wild rice
¼ cup ground flaxseed
¼ cup ground sesame seeds
2 tsp baking powder
½ tsp black pepper

- In a food processor, process all ingredients until smooth.
- Lightly oil a pan with coconut oil and heat over medium heat. Pour in pancake batter to desired pancake size and cook for about 5 minutes or until bubbles begin to appear. Flip and allow to cook for another 5 minutes.

salads

In general, since salads tend to be lower in carbohydrate, yet higher in minerals, they are usually best eaten later in the day, when the body doesn't require as much fuel (carbohydrate) but does need nutrition to rebuild and repair from the day's activities. For this reason I have one salad a day, always as dinner, or as part of dinner.

Thai Salad

MATTHEW KENNEY

A raw twist on a classic.

Time: 15 minutes • Makes 2 servings

2 handfuls mixed greens
½ cup finely diced pineapple
½ cup soaked, finely sliced sun-dried tomatoes
1 avocado, sliced
Sea salt
Freshly ground black pepper
½ red bell pepper, cut into long, thin strips
½ cup thinly sliced young coconut meat
½ cup chopped cashews
½ cup Creamy Thai Dressing (see p. 215)
Cilantro leaves, for garnish

- Place a handful of mixed greens in the center of each plate. Top with pineapple, sun-dried tomatoes, and avocado.
- Season with salt and pepper to taste. Top with red bell pepper, coconut, and cashews.
- Drizzle Creamy Thai Dressing generously over top just before serving. Garnish with cilantro leaves.

Beet Salad with Lemon Herb Cream Cheese

RAVENS' RESTAURANT, MENDOCINO, CALIFORNIA

Rich, earthy, full-flavored goodness. The chefs at Ravens' use a variety of beets from their garden, including Chioggia (also called candy-stripe) or yellow beets.

Time: 15 minutes active; 30 minutes to cook • Makes 4 servings

4 small garden beets
1 bunch of frisée or favorite greens (mesclun, arugula)

- Preheat oven to 450°F. Wash beets, then wrap in aluminum foil and roast in oven for 30 minutes. Remove from oven and allow to cool.
- When cool to the touch, slip off skins and slice.

DRESSING

3 tbsp Dijon mustard
¼ cup finely chopped shallots
½ cup white balsamic vinegar

2 cups olive oil
½ cup agave nectar
Salt to taste

- Mix all ingredients together.

LEMON HERB CREAM CHEESE

½ cup raw walnuts
Juice from ½ lemon (reserve second half, zest removed)

Lemon zest (add to taste)
1 clove garlic
Pinch of salt

- Place all ingredients in a food processor. Process until mixture resembles a coarse cream cheese. Add additional lemon juice if necessary and lemon zest for flavor.

To serve
- Arrange about one-quarter of the beets around the rim of a plate. Place one-quarter of the frisée in the center of the plate, then drizzle dressing over frisée and beets.
- Take two tablespoons: with one, scoop out some Lemon Herb Cream Cheese and with the other, form it into an ovoid shape and place on frisée.

Roasted Beet and Fennel Salad with Belgium Endive

MILLENNIUM RESTAURANT, SAN FRANCISCO, CALIFORNIA

A great winter salad. The rich dressing pairs well with the sweetness of the beets and bitterness of the endive.

Time: 15 minutes • Makes 2 servings

2 cups small diced beets
2 cups small diced fennel bulb
2–3 tsp olive oil
2 tsp balsamic vinegar
Juice of ½ Meyer lemon (optional)
Salt to taste
Black pepper to taste

- Blanch the beets and fennel for 3–4 minutes. Drain and toss with a small amount of olive oil and the balsamic vinegar.
- Roast on a non-stick baking mat or a parchment-lined sheet pan until al dente and glazed.
- Toss with Meyer lemon juice, if using. Adjust salt and pepper to taste.

To serve
6 Belgian endive spears per salad
Roasted beets and fennel mixture
Garlic-Green Peppercorn Dressing (see p. 212)
Grapefruit or mandarin orange segments, for garnish
Fresh tarragon and flat leaf parsley, for garnish

- For each salad, arrange endive around the perimeter of the plate. Fill each spear with the beet and fennel mixture.
- Drizzle the plate with 1–1 ½ ounces Garlic-Green Peppercorn Dressing.
- Garnish with grapefruit or mandarin orange segments, and a sprinkling of fresh tarragon and parsley leaves.

Roasted Vegetable Salad with Roasted Garlic Dressing

CANDLE 79, MANHATTAN, NEW YORK

Abigael Birrell, a Candle 79 chef, invented this luscious salad, full of roasted seasonal vegetables. She likes to serve it as a starter to a festive holiday dinner. It's also a good main course salad.

Time: 15 minutes active; 35–40 minutes to cook • Makes 4 servings

1 fennel bulb, trimmed and cut into bite-sized pieces
2 cups fingerling or new potatoes, cut into bite-sized pieces
1 cup baby turnips, peeled and cut into bite-sized pieces
2 medium-sized beets, peeled and cut into bite-sized pieces
2 medium apples, cored and sliced
1 tsp sea salt
Freshly ground black pepper
3 tbsp extra-virgin olive oil
Roasted Garlic Dressing (see p. 211)
2 bunches arugula, rinsed, trimmed, and stemmed
Toasted walnuts or pecans (optional)

- Preheat oven to 400°F.
- Toss the vegetables and apples with the salt, pepper, and olive oil in a large mixing bowl.
- Spread in a single layer on a baking sheet and bake until just tender, 35–40 minutes.
- Toss the vegetables with about 2 tbsp of Roasted Garlic Dressing to lightly coat the vegetables, and set aside.
- To serve the salad, arrange the arugula on 4 plates, then top with equal amounts of the warm vegetable mixture. Sprinkle with toasted walnuts or pecans, if desired, drizzle with a bit more dressing, and serve at once.

Shaved Zucchini and Sacha Inchi Salad

Refreshing yet filling.

Time: 10 minutes • Makes 4 servings

DRESSING

⅓ cup hemp oil (or Vega Antioxidant EFA oil)
2 tbsp fresh lemon juice
1 tsp coarse sea salt
½ tsp ground black pepper
¼ tsp dried crushed red pepper

- Mix oil, lemon juice, salt, black pepper, and crushed red pepper in a bowl. Set aside.

SALAD

2 pounds medium zucchini, trimmed
½ cup coarsely chopped fresh basil
¼ cup chopped sacha inchi
Salt and pepper to taste

- Using vegetable peeler, slice zucchini into ribbons, working from top to bottom of each zucchini. Put ribbons in large bowl.
- Add basil and chopped sacha inchi, then the dressing; toss to coat. Add salt and pepper, as much as desired.

Spicy Lentil Salad

Raw

BEETS LIVING FOODS CAFÉ, AUSTIN, TEXAS

Filling and protein-rich.

Time: 10 minutes • Makes 2 servings

2 tbsp minced onions
1 small clove of garlic, minced
¼ cup cilantro, finely chopped
2 medium tomatoes, finely chopped
½ tsp jalapeño, finely minced (or more for desired spice)
2 tsp lemon juice
1 cup sprouted lentils (½ cup before sprouting)
2 tsp apple cider vinegar
2 tsp olive oil
¼ tsp sea salt or to taste

- Place onions, garlic, cilantro, tomatoes, jalapeño, and lemon juice into a medium bowl and mix well.
- Add lentils, apple cider vinegar, and olive oil and mix. Add salt to taste.
- Store in the refrigerator.

Raw

Cumin-Style Cabbage Salad with Tart Green Apple

Unique and flavor-packed.

Time: 1 hour presoak; 15 minutes active • Makes 4–6 servings

½ medium green cabbage, sliced
    into thin strips
½ cup cashews, soaked in water
    for 1 hour
½ cup reserved cashew soak water
1 tbsp lime juice
½ tbsp balsamic vinegar

½ tsp ground cumin
1 clove garlic, peeled and
    mashed in a garlic press
1 tart green apple (such as
    Granny Smith variety),
    cut into matchsticks

- Place the cabbage in a large bowl and set aside.
- In a blender, combine the cashews, ½ cup soak water, lime juice, vinegar, cumin, and garlic and blend.
- Once the mixture is a smooth sauce, pour over the cabbage. Use clean hands to massage the sauce into the cabbage for a minute to help soften the cabbage slightly, into a slaw. Toss in the apple and serve.

Good Roots Salad with Coconut-Cumin Dressing

Surprisingly filling and energizing, this salad is packed with easily digestible carbohydrate. Be sure to peel all the vegetables before dicing and shredding.

Time: 10 minutes • Makes 4 servings

2 cups shredded beets (about
    2 medium)
2 cups shredded carrots (about
    4 medium)
4 cups diced jicama

2 tbsp pumpkin seeds
2 cups onion sprouts (about
    4 ounces in weight)
½ recipe Coconut-Cumin Dressing
    (see p. 215)

- Combine all ingredients and toss.

Raw

Dilled Spinach Salad with Avocado

Fresh tasting, filling, high in iron, and flavorful. If it's available, use fresh dill instead of dried. Add to taste.

Time: 10 minutes • Makes 2–4 servings

1 package (5 ounces) baby spinach leaves
1 beet, peeled and cut into large matchsticks
1 avocado, peeled and chopped
⅓ cup red onion, diced
2 tbsp hemp oil
1 tbsp balsamic vinegar
2 cloves garlic, pressed
1 tbsp dried dill
Salt and pepper to taste

- In a large bowl, combine the spinach, beet, avocado, and red onion.
- In a small bowl, whisk together the hemp oil, vinegar, pressed garlic, and dill. Add salt and pepper to taste.
- Just before serving, add the dressing to the salad and toss.

New Caesar Salad

With the distinctive flavor of a traditional Caesar salad, but with no cholesterol.

Time: 15 minutes • Makes 4 servings (1 cup of dressing)

DRESSING

¼ cup cashews
¼ cup water
¼ cup olive oil
2 ½ tbsp red wine vinegar
3 tbsp lemon juice
3 large cloves garlic
1 ½ tsp miso paste
3 tbsp wakame flakes
1 tsp Dijon mustard

• Blend all ingredients together.

SALAD

3–4 whole romaine lettuce hearts, torn into bite-sized pieces
Rustic Sweet Onion Flatbread (see p. 186) or flax crackers
½ ounce dulse strips, cut into small pieces
Freshly cracked black pepper, to taste

• Toss the lettuce with several spoonfuls of dressing in a large bowl (use as much dressing as desired). Place dressed greens on a plate along with a couple of pieces of Rustic Sweet Onion Flatbread or flax crackers and sprinkle with a few dulse strips. Generously adorn with some freshly cracked pepper.

Raw

Summertime Chef Salad

Fresh and light, this is a simple summertime staple.

Time: 10 minutes • Makes 4–6 servings

4–6 large handfuls mixed baby greens or chopped romaine lettuce
2 cups fresh white corn kernels (about 2 ears)
1 ½ cups grape tomatoes, halved
2 cups cucumber, thinly sliced
½ cup red onion, thinly sliced
4 cups jicama, cut into large matchsticks
1–2 avocados, cut into chunks
Dressing of choice

- For each serving, create a bed of greens, then place each of the other vegetables in a small mound around the plate for a decorative presentation. Drizzle with dressing of choice.

Summer Chopped Salad

TAL RONNEN

This is super-easy—a foolproof recipe—but you should make it right before you serve it. Chopped salads can get soggy if they sit around. Kids go crazy for this because of all the great flavors and textures.

Time: 20 minutes • Makes 4 servings

¼ pound green beans, cut into 1-inch pieces
5 radishes, finely diced
Dash of agave nectar
¼ English cucumber, finely diced
12 red and yellow cherry tomatoes, quartered
Kernels from 2 ears raw sweet corn
1 avocado, diced
1 cup baby arugula
1 shallot, minced
1 tsp minced fresh basil
1 tsp minced fresh oregano
Vinaigrette (see p. 214)
1 tsp freshly squeezed lemon juice

- Blanch the green beans in boiling water for 30 seconds, then chill in an ice bath. In the same boiling water, blanch the radishes for 20 seconds, then chill in an ice bath sweetened with a dash of agave nectar.
- Place all of the ingredients except for the Vinaigrette and lemon juice in a large bowl.
- Drizzle with the Vinaigrette and toss to coat. Sprinkle the lemon juice on top just before serving.

Watercress Salad with Roasted Beets

Unique and original flavor sets this nutrient-packed salad apart.

Time: 10 minutes; 1 hour to cool • Makes 4 starter salads

GINGERED BEETS

3 beets, washed and peeled
1 cup apple cider vinegar
2 tsp whole black peppercorns
2-inch piece of peeled ginger, cut into thin slices
¼ cup palm sugar

SALAD

2 bunches watercress, washed and de-stemmed
1–2 tbsp sesame seeds (black or white)
¼ cup Sweet Mustard Dressing (see p. 213)
Sesame seeds, for sprinkling

- Slice the beets into thin rounds and place in a large canning or heatproof jar.
- Pour the vinegar, peppercorns, ginger, and palm sugar into a small saucepan, and bring to a boil.
- Pour the hot mixture over the beets, seal jar, and place in the refrigerator. Beets may be enjoyed as soon as they have cooled (about 1 hour) or will keep in a closed, refrigerated container for up to 1 month.
- To prepare the salad, toss the watercress with the Sweet Mustard Dressing and divide onto serving plates.
- Place the beets on top of the greens, and sprinkle with sesame seeds.

Mexican Salad Bowl

Traditional Mexican salad.

Time: 10 minutes • Makes 4 servings

2 large handfuls baby salad greens
  or chopped romaine lettuce
1 cup cooked black beans
1 cup jicama, cubed
2 cups shredded carrots (about
  3 carrots)

1 cup sweet corn kernels
  (about one ear)
¼ cup chopped green onion

- In a large bowl, toss the vegetables with the dressing of your choice and serve.

Wilted Chard Salad with Lima Beans

Can be served as a meal.

Time: 10 minutes • Makes 2–4 servings

1 tbsp coconut oil
1 leek, white and light green parts,
  sliced thin
2 cloves garlic, minced
¼ tsp sea salt, or to taste
1 large bunch Swiss chard, stems
  removed, sliced into ½-inch strips

2 tsp balsamic vinegar
1 cup fresh or frozen lima beans,
  blanched for 2 minutes
¼ tsp red pepper flakes

- Heat the oil in a large skillet over medium heat until melted. Add the leek and the garlic and sauté for 2 minutes, stirring often, until the leeks have softened.
- Add the salt, Swiss chard, balsamic vinegar, lima beans, and red pepper flakes, and toss to combine.
- Cover the pan, reduce heat to medium-low, and cook for 4–5 minutes, until the chard has wilted. Remove from heat and serve immediately.

South of the Border Coleslaw

A fresh take on coleslaw.

Time: 15 minutes active; cashew soak time • Makes 4–6 servings

½ cup cashews, soaked in water for 1–2 hours
½ cup cashew soak water
2 tsp apple cider vinegar
2 large Medjool dates, pits removed
½ packed cup fresh cilantro, plus more for garnish
½ tsp sea salt
8 cups finely shredded green cabbage (shredded as thinly as possible)
1 cup shredded carrots

- When cashews are soaked and soft, place in a blender with water, vinegar, dates, cilantro, and salt. Blend until smooth and creamy (this may take a couple of minutes).
- In a bowl, mix together the cabbage and carrots. Pour the blended mixture on top and toss until well coated.
- Garnish with additional cilantro, if desired.

Dandelion Salad with Sun-Dried Tomatoes and Lentil Dressing

Flavorful sun-dried tomatoes combined with the bitterness of the dandelion greens give this salad special qualities. Lovers of bitter greens can substitute the mixed greens for additional dandelion.

Time: 5 minutes active; tomato presoak time • Makes 2–4 servings

2 heaping handfuls dandelion greens (about ½ bunch), trimmed and
    cut in half lengthwise
2 heaping handfuls baby mixed greens
⅔ cup sun-dried tomatoes, soaked 30 minutes in warm water until soft,
    sliced into ¼-inch strips
1 tbsp minced shallot
½ recipe Lentil Dressing (see p. 214)
⅓ cup cooked green lentils
Freshly cracked pepper

- In a large bowl, combine the greens, sun-dried tomatoes, and shallot. Pour the lentil dressing on top and toss thoroughly.
- To serve, top with ⅓ cup lentils and freshly cracked pepper.

Hemp Seed Kale Salad

Classic nutrient-rich, alkaline-forming salad at its best.

Time: 10 minutes • Makes 2–4 servings

1 large bunch of curly or latigo kale
3 green onions, minced (white parts only)
½ cup diced crimini mushrooms (optional)
1 tbsp red wine vinegar
1 tbsp miso paste
2 tbsp hemp oil
¼ tsp garlic powder
⅓ cup hemp seeds
1 red bell pepper, finely diced

- Wash and dry the kale thoroughly. Strip the stems away from the kale leaves and discard. Place the kale leaves in a large bowl, tearing apart any large pieces.
- Add the green onions, mushrooms, red wine vinegar, miso paste, hemp oil, and garlic powder.
- Use your hands to massage the ingredients into the kale for about 2 minutes, or until kale and mushrooms have softened slightly.
- Add the hemp seeds and bell pepper and toss thoroughly.

Quick Kale Avocado Salad

CHAD SARNO

This is a wonderful way to enjoy the mighty kale. Many are unfamiliar with raw kale, but working with this method of softening the kale with the other ingredients makes it not only much easier to digest but also incredibly delicious. Serve this recipe with your favorite cooked whole grain and a handful of raw or toasted seeds/nuts for a great protein-packed alkalizing meal.

Time: 10 minutes • Makes 2 servings

1 head kale, shredded (any variety is great)
1 large tomato, or red bell pepper, diced
1 ½ avocado, chopped
3 tbsp flaxseed oil
2 tbsp red onion, green onion, or leeks, finely diced
1 lemon, juiced
1 tsp sea salt
Diced fresh chilies or pinch of cayenne (optional)

- In large mixing bowl toss all ingredients together, squeezing as you mix to "wilt" the kale and cream the avocado. Serve immediately. This dish is also great if you want to use chard, collards, broccoli leaves, spinach, or any combination of these instead of kale.

Chinese Chopped Salad

A healthy makeover of a Chinese chicken salad, this fresh preparation offers substantial amounts of protein of the plant-based variety.

Time: 15 minutes • Makes 4 servings

DRESSING

1 ½ tbsp yacon syrup or agave nectar
1 ½ tbsp ume plum vinegar
1 ½ tbsp apple cider vinegar
1 tbsp + 1 tsp fresh ginger, grated
1 whole red jalapeño pepper, minced (with or without seeds)
¼ cup hemp oil or olive oil
2 tbsp fresh squeezed orange juice
¼ cup sesame seeds

- Combine all the dressing ingredients, except 2 tbsp of sesame seeds, in a blender, blending until as creamy as possible. Stir in the remaining sesame seeds by hand and refrigerate until ready to use.

SALAD

5 cups Chinese cabbage, shredded
5 cups romaine lettuce, shredded
¼ cup scallions, white and green parts
1 cup snow peas or sugar snap peas
2 cups mung bean sprouts
¾ cup chopped roasted sacha inchi seeds (or almonds)
½ cup dried goldenberries (optional)

- In a large bowl, chop and combine all salad ingredients, except for the sacha inchi seeds and goldenberries.
- Toss with dressing just before serving. Sprinkle with sacha inchi seeds and goldenberries.

Chopped Garden Salad

This is a really flexible recipe. Pick a dressing of your choice or just do simple oil and vinegar.

Time: 15 minutes • Makes 2 very large dinner salads or 4–6 side salads

1 large head romaine lettuce
2 carrots
1 large cucumber (if organic, do not peel)
2 large radishes
1 stalk celery
1 cup onion sprouts (or use another kind of sprout)
¼ cup sunflower seeds
2 tbsp hemp seeds (optional)
Salad dressing of choice

- Chop the lettuce, carrots, cucumber, radishes, and celery finely.
- Toss together in a large bowl with sprouts, sunflower seeds, and hemp seeds.
- Add dressing, if desired, just before serving.

Raw

Asian Vegetable Noodle Salad

A raw twist on an ancient classic.

Time: 10 minutes • Makes 2–4 servings

DRESSING

1 tbsp + 1 tsp hemp oil or olive oil
2 tsp sesame oil
2 tsp miso paste
2 ½ tbsp yacon syrup
2 tbsp balsamic vinegar

- Combine all the ingredients in a jar and mix well.

SALAD

6 large zucchinis, peeled with a vegetable peeler into long strips
2 carrots, peeled with a vegetable peeler into long strips
1 package of kelp noodles, drained (optional)
2 green onions
½ jalapeño, deseeded and minced
¼ cup chopped sacha inchi or chopped almonds
Cilantro leaves, for garnish (optional)

- Toss together the salad vegetables in a large bowl, mix in the dressing, and top with sacha inchi or almonds and cilantro.

Asian Carrot Avocado Salad

A quick and easy salad with an exquisite balance of Asian-influenced flavor. An all-time favorite recipe!

Time: 10 minutes • Makes 3–4 servings

DRESSING

2 tbsp flaxseed oil
3 tbsp lime juice
2 tsp ume plum vinegar
1 tbsp fresh ginger, grated
1 tbsp ground coriander
1 tbsp agave nectar

- In a food processor, blend oil, lime juice, miso, ginger, coriander, and agave nectar.

SALAD

4 cups grated carrots
½ cup cilantro, chopped
½ cup parsley, chopped
1 green onion, sliced (white and 1 inch of green parts)
½ cup raw sesame seeds, with 2 tbsp set aside
1 medium avocado, chopped

- Grate carrots and toss in a large bowl with cilantro, parsley, green onion, and sesame seeds (reserving 2 tbsp of seeds). Set aside.

To serve
- Pour dressing over salad, and toss well. Gently fold in avocado, and sprinkle reserved sesame seeds on top before serving.

Candied Grapefruit Salad

AMANDA COHEN

This is our way to make salad more fun. Start by preparing the grapefruit so the candy glaze can dry while you work on the rest of the recipe. You'll need a candy thermometer to test when the palm sugar's ready for dipping, and a sturdy piece of floral foam or Styrofoam heavy enough to hold the skewers upright while the grapefruit dries.

Time: 1 hour • Makes 4 servings

8 grapefruit segments with the peel removed, but as much of the pith (the white skin beneath the peel) left on as possible

8 eight-inch bamboo skewers
3 cups palm sugar
½ cup water

- Push the skewers through the bottom of the grapefruit segments until they're about halfway in.
- In a heavy stockpot, bring the sugar and water to 250°F. Insert the thermometer just to check temperature, then remove.
- Dip each skewered piece of grapefruit in the hot sugar and coat each thoroughly.
- Stick the bottom ends of the skewers into the foam and let them dry until hard.

DRESSING

¼ cup grapefruit juice
2 tbsp grapefruit zest
2 tbsp lemon juice
1 tbsp finely minced shallot

½ tsp Dijon mustard
¾ cup extra-virgin olive oil
2 tsp salt
¼ tsp pepper

- Blend everything but the oil in a blender, and then slowly stream in the oil. Add salt and pepper to taste.

SALAD

4 cups mixed greens
¼ ripe avocado, cubed
3 tbsp toasted sliced almonds

- Mix the greens with the salad dressing, and toss in the avocado and almonds. Divide among 4 plates. Put two grapefruit skewers on each plate.

Cream of Asparagus Soup

Tal Ronnen

Tal says, "When I lived in Virginia, asparagus was one of the only locally fresh vegetables you could find in spring. This recipe is versatile: If you can't find nice asparagus, use broccoli to make cream of broccoli instead. As in a lot of my recipes, cashew cream stands in for dairy here and makes for an equally rich, delicious dish."

Time: 1 hour, 15 minutes prep   •   Makes 6 servings

Sea salt
3 tbsp extra-virgin olive oil
1 large bunch asparagus, ends trimmed,
    cut into 2-inch pieces
2 stalks celery, chopped
1 large onion, chopped
2 quarts faux chicken or vegetable stock
    (try Better Than Bouillon brand)

1 bay leaf
1 cup Thick Cashew Cream
    (see p. 209) + 6 tsp, for garnish
Freshly ground black pepper
2 cups fresh baby spinach
Microgreens, for garnish

- Place a large stockpot over medium heat. Sprinkle the bottom with a pinch of salt and heat for 1 minute. Add the oil and heat for 30 seconds, being careful not to let it smoke. This will create a non-stick effect.
- Add the asparagus, celery, and onion and sauté for 6–10 minutes, until the celery is just soft. Add the stock and bay leaf, bring to a boil, then reduce the heat and simmer for 30 minutes. Add the Thick Cashew Cream and simmer for an additional 10 minutes. Remove and discard the bay leaf. Season to taste with salt and pepper.
- Working in batches, pour the soup into a blender, cover the lid with a towel (the hot liquid tends to erupt), and blend on high. Add the spinach to the last batch and continue blending until smooth. Pour the soup into a large bowl and stir to incorporate the spinach batch. Ladle into bowls. Garnish each bowl with microgreens and a teaspoon of Thick Cashew Cream.

Consommé: Tomato Water, Merlot-Pickled Onions, Avocado, and Mint

Chad Sarno

Elaborate but ideal if you want to be fancy. If you plan to use one of the garnish options to dress up the meal, begin its preparation the night before or a day ahead so it's ready in time.

Time: 20 minutes active; 1 hour sit time for tomatoes • Makes 6 servings

12 vine tomatoes, chopped (mixed heirloom tomatoes preferred)
2 tsp sea salt
2 cloves garlic, sliced
1 tsp fresh chili, chopped
2 tbsp merlot vinegar (or aged sherry vinegar as substitution)
Mint leaves, torn, for garnish

- To release the natural water from the tomato, toss the chopped tomatoes with the sea salt, then massage the tomatoes to release water.
- Add sliced garlic, chopped chili, and merlot vinegar to the tomatoes. Allow to sit for ½–1 hour or so for flavors to marry in room temperature. During this time the tomato water will begin to drain off—help the process by regularly massaging the tomatoes.
- Saving the liquid for the broth, strain off tomato liquid with either a fine mesh strainer or a sprouting bag. (For a clear water, allow the mixture to hang in the sprouting bag so that gravity releases the clear tomato water ... for faster production, use the fine mesh strainer instead.) Store the tomato pulp for a future dish.
- Serve chilled and garnished with Wine Pickled Onions (recipe on the next page), torn mint leaves, and avocado balls. Alternatively, garnish with Cucumber-Cress Sorbet (recipe on the next page).

WINE-PICKLED ONIONS

2 red onions, peeled, and sliced paper-thin on mandolin
½ cup red wine or merlot vinegar
3 tbsp agave syrup
Pinch of coarse sea salt
Pinch of cracked black pepper

- Toss all ingredients well, and gently massage. Allow to pickle for a few hours to overnight. Store in a jar and refrigerate; they will keep for up to 2 weeks.

CUCUMBER-CRESS SORBET (OPTIONAL SERVICE SUGGESTION)

½ cup cashews, soaked
1 avocado, removed from skin
½ cup watercress
½ cup cucumber, peeled
2 tbsp agave syrup
1 tbsp lemon juice
1 clove garlic
1 tsp sea salt
¼ cup water

- In high-speed blender, blend all ingredients until smooth. Either pour it into your choice of sorbet maker, following manufacturer's instructions, or line a square container with plastic wrap, then pour in blended mixture.
- Freeze overnight, pop the frozen block out the following day, slice it in strips, and put them through a single- or double-gear juicer, using the solid plate instead of the juicing screen, for a delicious sorbet!
- Serve a small quenelle with each bowl of consommé.

Black Bean Soup

CANDLE 79, MANHATTAN, NEW YORK

The day before you want to make this soup, soak your beans overnight in the refrigerator. It cuts down on the cooking time and makes them more digestible.

Time: 20 minutes prep; 45 minutes to cook • Makes 6 servings

2 tbsp extra-virgin olive oil
1 cup diced celery
1 cup diced yellow onion
¼ cup sliced leeks, trimmed and cleaned
1 cup diced zucchini
2 cloves garlic, minced
1 dried chipotle pepper
2 cups black beans, soaked overnight
1 bay leaf
1 tsp sea salt
12 cups filtered water
4 tbsp fresh cilantro, chopped
1 tsp fresh oregano, chopped
Chopped tomatoes, sliced avocado, tofu sour cream for garnish

- In a 4-quart pot, heat olive oil on medium heat. Add celery, onion, leeks, zucchini, garlic, and chipotle pepper. Sauté vegetables for 10–15 minutes or until they become translucent and very soft.
- Add black beans, bay leaf, salt, and filtered water. Cover pot, reduce heat to low, and allow to cook for 45 minutes or until the beans are cooked and all the vegetables have almost disappeared into the soup. The beans should be creamy in texture.
- Remove the bay leaf and divide the soup. Allow it to cool slightly and purée half in blender, beans too. Be very careful not to place the hot soup in the blender or else it will end up everywhere!
- Add puréed mixture to reserved soup. Stir in cilantro and oregano, and return to heat for about 5–10 minutes to reheat.
- Garnish with chopped tomatoes, sliced avocado, and tofu sour cream, or enjoy as is!

Tomato Soup

A plant-based twist on a classic creamy soup.

Time: 5 minutes (once Marinara/Pizza Sauce and UnMotza Macadamia Cheese are made) • Makes 1 serving

4 tbsp tomato sauce or Marinara/Pizza
    Sauce (see p. 206)
1–2 tbsp UnMotza Macadamia Cheese
    Sauce (see p. 206)
4 tbsp chopped tomato
2 tbsp chopped cucumber, red bell
    pepper, zucchini
1 tbsp red onion
2 tbsp sunflower sprouts

½ clove of garlic
1 tsp each sea salt and dried oregano
1 tbsp extra-virgin olive oil
1 tsp apple cider vinegar
Pinch of black pepper
1 cup of warm or hot water
Optional: 1 tsp nutritional flakes,
    chopped cilantro, or parsley,
    or all three

- Combine all ingredients in a bowl and eat as is, or combine in a blender and blend until smooth.

Curry Soup

Rich and filling.

Time: 10 minutes (once UnMotza Macadamia Cheese Sauce is made)
Makes 1 serving

4 tbsp UnMotza Macadamia Cheese
    Sauce (see p. 206)
2 tbsp chopped red bell pepper
4 tbsp chopped zucchini
1 tbsp red onion
3 tbsp chopped celery
½ clove of garlic
2 tbsp sunflower sprouts

1 tsp each sun dried sea salt and
    curry powder
¼ tsp turmeric powder
1 tbsp first cold pressed coconut oil
1 tsp apple cider vinegar
Pinch of black pepper
1 cup warm or hot water
Optional: 1 tsp nutritional flakes

- In a blender, combine all ingredients, except UnMotza Macadamia Cheese Sauce, and blend until smooth.
- Pour soup into a bowl and pour UnMotza Macadamia Cheese Sauce on top.

Raw

Very Green Raw Soup

JIVAMUKTEA CAFÉ, MANHATTAN, NEW YORK

This soup is like a green juice, with all the whole food fiber benefits.

Time: 5 minutes prep • Makes 1 serving

Bowl of mixed lettuce greens
4 cherry tomatoes
½ apple
1 tsp spirulina powder (optional)

1 tbsp olive oil
1 tsp lemon or lime juice
Salt and pepper to taste
Approx 1 cup water

- Place all ingredients into a blender or food processor. Add just enough water to blend ingredients into a creamy consistency and serve cold.

Raw

Spinach Cream Soup

CRUDESSENCE, MONTREAL, QUEBEC

Creamy and filling, this soup is chlorophyll-rich.

Time: 5 minutes • Makes 4 servings

¼ cup shelled pistachios
⅛ cup pine nuts
1¼ cups spinach
⅔ cup avocado
¼ cup lemon juice
3 cups water

⅓ cup red onions
1 tsp sea salt
½ tsp ground black pepper
1 small clove garlic
1 tbsp dried rosemary

- Place all ingredients into a blender and blend thoroughly until the texture is smooth and creamy. Serve cold.

Raw

Chilled Summer Greens and Avocado Soup
with Truffled Cashew Sour Cream

MILLENNIUM RESTAURANT, SAN FRANCISCO, CALIFORNIA

Sophisticated and nutritious.

Time: 10 minutes • Makes 4 servings

3–4 medium avocados (ripe)

2 scallions

1 cup diced seeded cucumber

2 cups watercress or arugula

Juice of 2 lemons

1 ½ cups water

Salt and pepper to taste

- In a blender, combine all ingredients and purée. Adjust salt and pepper to taste.
- Serve or chill covered with wrap on top of the soup to keep it from oxidizing. Do not store more than 2 hours.
- Serve each portion with fresh herbs of choice, a drizzle of a peppery-grassy olive oil (Posolivo, Scabicia Tuscan or Sevillano, or Arbequenia varietal oil), and 2 tsp of Cashew–Truffle Oil Cream (see p. 208).

Raw

Cool Cantaloupe Soup

Simple summer refreshment. Almost an applesauce-like texture.

Time: 10 minutes • Makes 2–4 servings

4 cups cantaloupe flesh (about 1 medium)

2 tbsp fresh lemon juice

2 tbsp fresh lime juice

- In a blender, combine all ingredients and blend until smooth. Chill before serving.

Chilled Cream of Beet Soup

Sweet beets combine with creamy avocados for this alluring, satisfying, and not to mention stunningly colored soup. This soup has great healthy benefits too. It is vegan, gluten free, and cholesterol free.

Time: 10 minutes prep; 1 hour to roast • Makes 4 servings

4 medium beets
1 avocado, chopped
1 lime, juiced
2 cups water
3 tbsp hemp seeds
1 tbsp ground coriander
¼ tsp sea salt
Fresh cilantro leaves and black pepper, for garnish (optional)

- Heat the oven to 350°F. Trim the beets and remove stems and end. Individually wrap each beet in tin foil. Roast for 1 hour and allow to cool completely.
- Using a paper towel, rub off the beet skins. Chop coarsely.
- Place the cooled beets, avocado, lime juice, water, hemp seeds, coriander, and sea salt in a blender. Blend until completely smooth.
- Place soup into refrigerator, and allow to chill for a minimum of 30 minutes.
- Pour into serving bowls and sprinkle with cilantro and black pepper, if desired.

Chilled Cucumber Avocado Soup

HORIZONS, PHILADELPHIA, PENNSYLVANIA

Time: 15 minutes prep; 1 hour to chill • Makes 6 servings

8 cucumbers, peeled and seeded
¼ cup chopped onion
1 bunch fresh cilantro, leaves only
½ cup fresh mint leaves (packed)
2 limes, juiced
1 ripe avocado
1 clove garlic
2 tbsp olive oil
2 tsp salt
2 tsp pepper
1 tsp organic palm sugar
¼ cup vegan mayo (preferably veganaise)
½ tsp Dijon mustard
Toasted pumpkin seeds, for garnish
Cumin oil (olive oil with ground cumin, lightly heated then cooled)

- Purée all ingredients in a food processor, except pumpkin seeds and cumin oil, adding in enough water to reach the consistency you like. It should be fairly thick, but adjust to your liking. Let chill for at least 1 hour.
- Serve chilled and garnish with toasted pumpkin seeds and cumin oil.

Lentil Soup with Wilted Spinach

A filling protein- and chlorophyll-rich soup.

Time: 40 minutes • Makes 4 servings

1 tbsp coconut oil
2 large cloves garlic, minced
2 cups vegetable broth
1 cup dry lentils, rinsed thoroughly

1 bay leaf
2 tbsp fresh lemon juice
2 cups packed baby spinach leaves
Salt and pepper to taste

- In a large soup pot, heat the coconut oil over medium heat. Add the garlic, and cook for 1 minute until garlic is fragrant and begins to turn golden.
- Pour in the vegetable broth, and add the lentils and bay leaf. Raise the heat to bring to a boil, then reduce heat to maintain a simmer.
- Cook, uncovered, for about 30 minutes, until lentils are just tender, adding more water if necessary to maintain a broth around the legumes.
- Stir in the lemon juice and the spinach and cook for 2 minutes longer, or until spinach has turned bright green and has wilted. Season with salt and pepper to taste and serve warm.

Chilled Carrot Ginger Soup

The ginger in this recipe is very light. Ginger lovers can easily up the quantity.

Time: 5 minutes • Makes 2–4 servings (4 cups)

3 cups carrot juice
1 avocado (peeled and pitted)
1 tbsp minced fresh ginger
2 tsp miso paste

- Combine all ingredients in a blender and blend until smooth. Serve chilled or slightly warmed.

Young Coconut Soup

Delicately seasoned. Add more jalapeño or ginger for a spicier taste.

Time: 10 minutes • Makes 2–4 servings (4 cups)

2 cups young coconut meat (about
   2–4 young coconuts)
2 cups young coconut water
4 dice-sized cubes of peeled fresh ginger

2 tsp fresh lime juice
1 tsp yacon syrup
1 jalapeño pepper, de-seeded
¼ tsp sea salt

- Combine all ingredients in a blender and blend until smooth and creamy. Serve chilled or at room temperature.

Fresh and Creamy Tomato Basil Soup

This soup is best when made during the peak tomato season—summer—for maximum flavor. If tomatoes are not in their prime or simply not sweet enough, add a touch more yacon syrup to balance the acidity.

Time: 10 minutes active; 1–2 hours presoak; 30 minutes to chill • Makes 2 ½ cups

3 medium tomatoes
½ cup raw cashews, presoaked in water
   (1–2 hours)
1 ½ tbsp yacon syrup
2 tbsp olive oil

1 ½ tbsp grated white onion
¼ cup shredded fresh basil + extra
   for garnish
¼ + ⅛ tsp sea salt
Fresh black pepper to taste

- Cut the tomatoes in half. Remove and discard all the seeds, then coarsely chop the remaining tomato and place in blender.
- Drain the cashews, reserving ½ cup water, and place in a blender.
- Combine all remaining ingredients in a blender, including the reserved soak water, and blend until smooth and creamy. If necessary, add more water to achieve desired texture.
- Allow soup to chill in refrigerator for 30 minutes or longer before serving.

Purée of Turnip Soup

A comforting holistic soup made from the delicious yet often forgotten turnip.

Time: 40 minutes • Makes 4 servings

2 tbsp coconut oil
1 medium yellow onion, chopped
2 large cloves garlic, minced
3–4 turnips (about 1 pound), chopped into 1-inch pieces
1 medium sweet potato (about ½ pound), peeled and chopped into 1-inch pieces
2 ½ cups vegetable broth
1 cup unsweetened almond milk
¼ tsp salt, or to taste
½ tsp black pepper

- Heat a large saucepan over medium heat. Melt the coconut oil, and add the onions and garlic. Sauté for 3–5 minutes or until onions begin to turn translucent.
- Add the turnips and the sweet potato and sauté for 2 minutes longer. Pour in the vegetable broth and almond milk. Bring to a boil, then reduce heat and simmer for 20–25 minutes, or until turnips and potatoes are tender.
- Transfer soup contents to a blender, and purée until completely smooth (blend in a couple of small batches, if necessary).
- Pour soup back into pot and reduce at a low simmer for 5 minutes longer. Add salt to taste and black pepper.

Puréed White Bean Soup

Simple and warming.

Time: 25 minutes • Makes 4–6 servings

1 tbsp coconut oil
2 leeks, white and light green parts sliced thin
1 tsp fresh thyme
3 tbsp lemon juice
30 ounces cooked white beans (fresh or canned)
2 ½ cups water
¼ cup cashews
1 tsp palm sugar
Salt and freshly ground black pepper, to taste
Fresh thyme leaves and freshly cracked pepper, for garnish

- In a large saucepan, heat the coconut oil, leeks, and thyme over medium-high heat for 2 minutes, or until the leeks are just softened.
- Transfer mixture to a blender and add lemon juice, beans, water, cashews, sugar, a pinch of salt, and a generous amount of black pepper. Blend on high for several minutes until completely smooth.
- Transfer back to the saucepan and simmer at medium-low heat for about 15 minutes, stirring occasionally. Do not overcook or soup will become too thick—add additional water if needed.
- Season with additional salt if desired, and garnish each bowl lightly with fresh thyme leaves and freshly cracked pepper before serving.

Stuffed Mushrooms

Raw

KARYN'S FRESH CORNER CAFÉ, CHICAGO, ILLINOIS

Time: 15 minutes active; 6 hours to soak; 1–2 hours to sit • Makes 6 servings

2 cups almonds (soaked)
20–30 button mushrooms
Bit of olive oil and salt (to massage
   on mushrooms)
½ yellow or green pepper
½ red pepper

2 stalks celery
3 cloves garlic
¼ cup olive oil
1 tsp salt

- Soak the almonds for 6 hours in purified water, drain, and rinse. Set aside.
- De-stem the mushrooms. Massage the caps very gently with a bit of oil and salt and let sit for 1–2 hours.
- Purée the almonds, peppers, celery, garlic, olive oil, and salt in food processor. Stuff pâté mixture into the mushroom caps.

Arame Sesame Brown Rice

RAVENS' RESTAURANT, MENDOCINO, CALIFORNIA

A Japanese macrobiotic-inspired classic.

Time: 5 minutes (once rice is cooked) • Makes 4 servings

2 tbsp sesame oil
½ cup bell peppers, diced
3 tbsp toasted arame

4 cups cooked rice
2 scallions, chopped, for garnish
2 tbsp sesame seeds, for garnish

- In saucepan, heat the sesame oil, then add the peppers and arame and sauté for 1 minute on medium-high heat.
- Add rice and stir well until heated thoroughly.
- Garnish with scallions and sesame seeds.

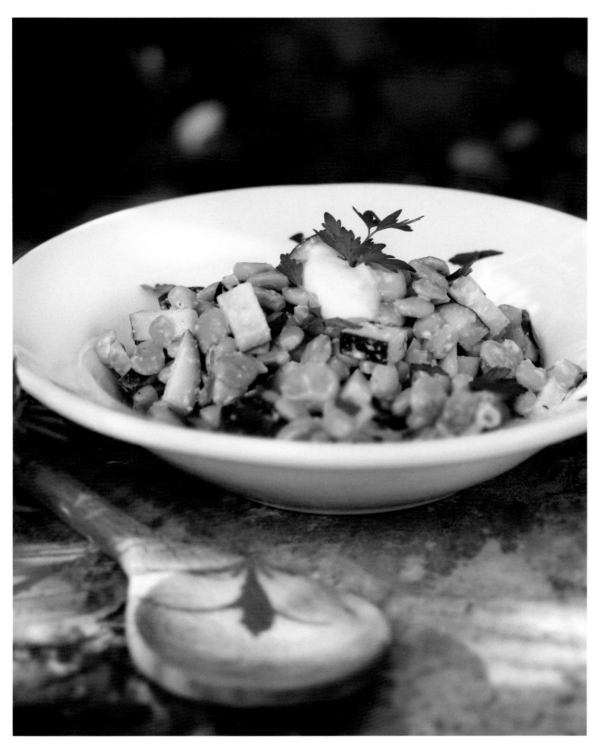

Summertime Succotash with Creamy Rosemary-Garlic Sauce (page 222)

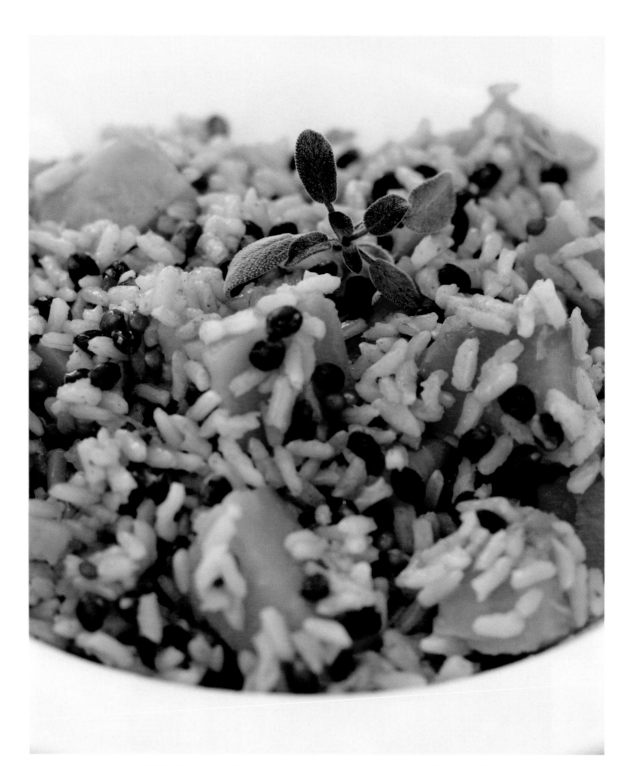

Wild Rice with Kabocha Squash and Sage Butter (page 238)

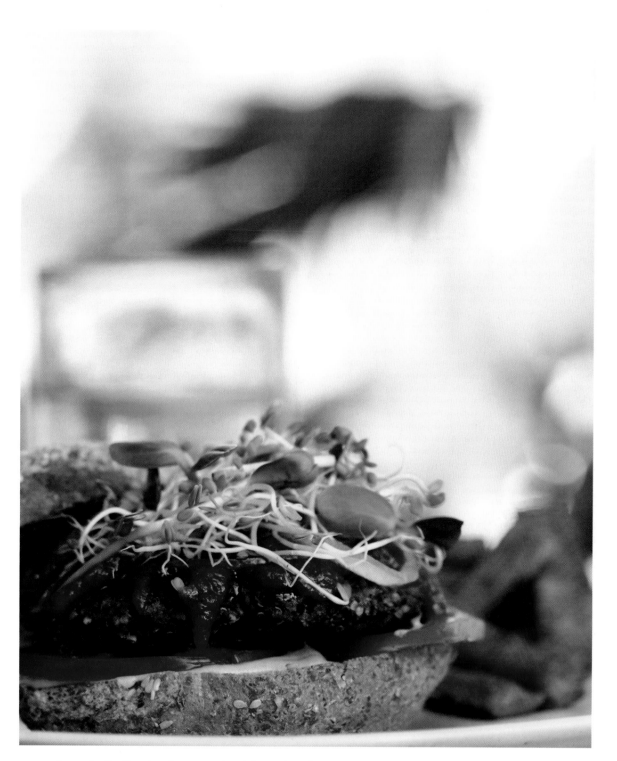

Portobello Patties (page 247) with Garlic Thyme Sweet Potato Oven Fries (page 179)

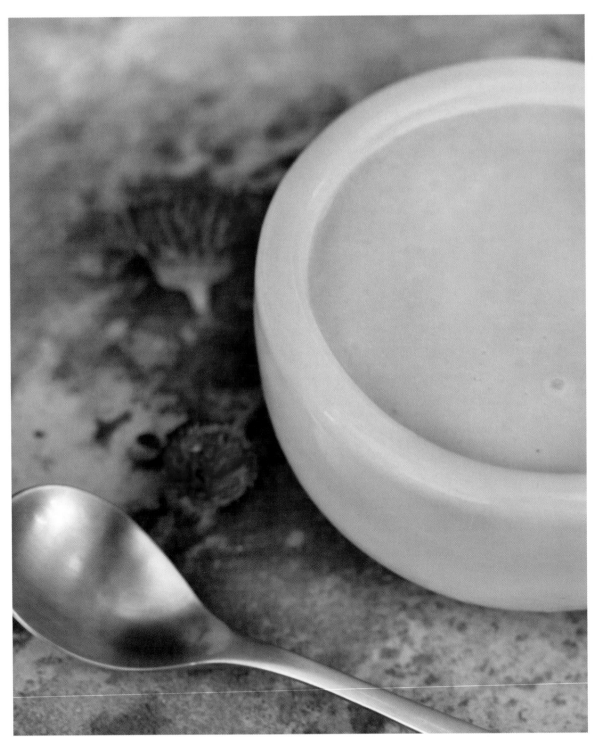

Young Coconut Soup (page 175)

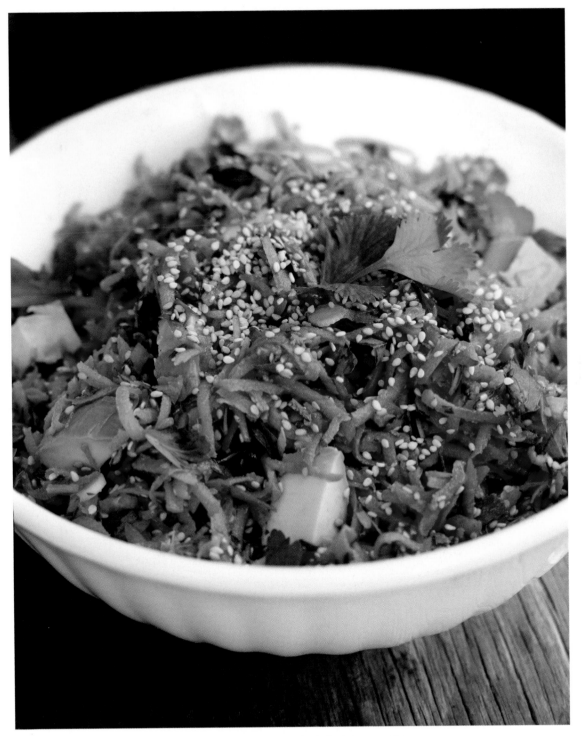

Asian Carrot Avocado Salad (page 163)

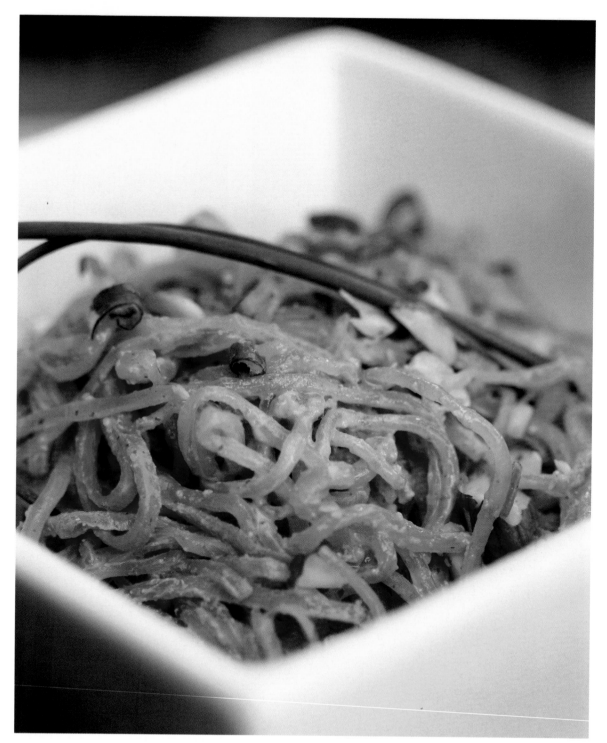
Almond Noodles with Carrots and Wakame (page 190)

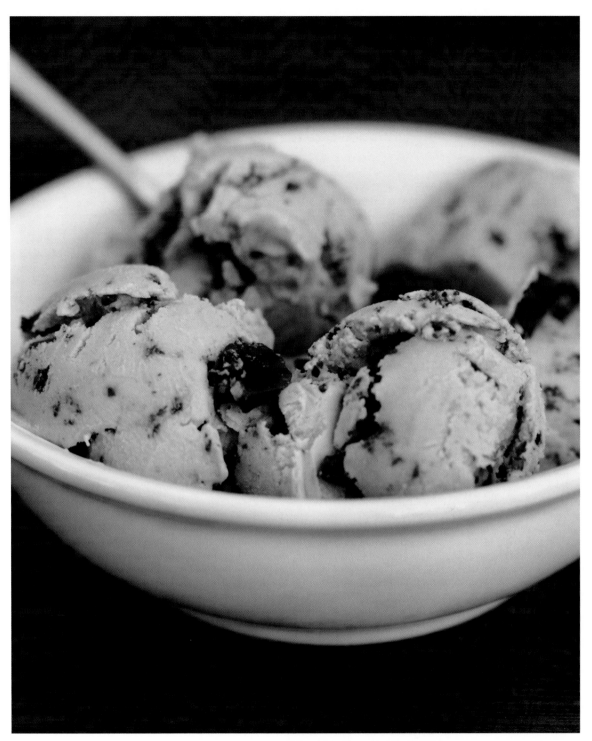

Chocolate Chip–Maple Maca Ice Cream (page 285)

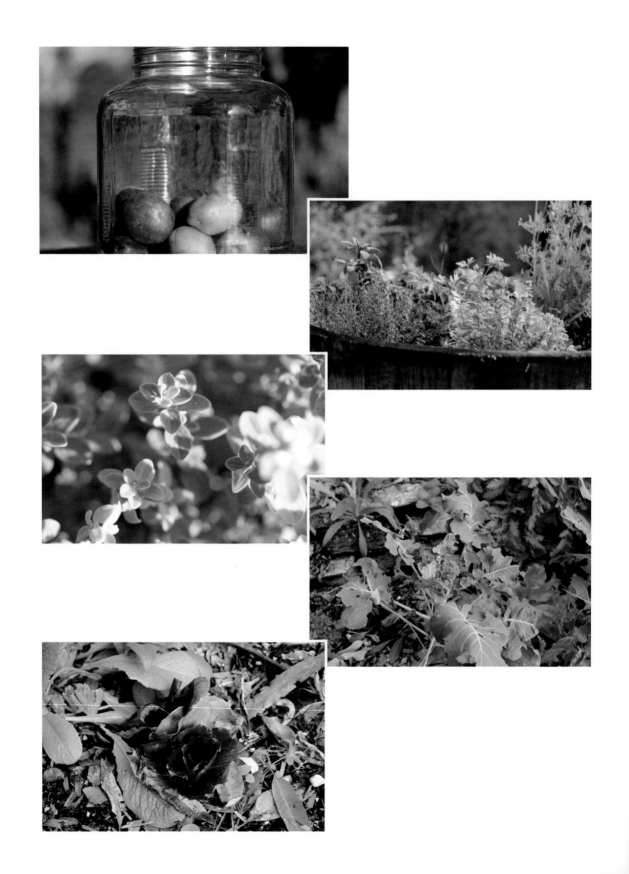

Mashed Kabocha Squash with Toasted Coconut

This delicious recipe makes a great side dish.

Time: 10 minutes • Makes 4 servings

¼ cup shredded coconut
1 pound cooked kabocha squash
3 tbsp light coconut milk
Salt and pepper, to taste

- In a pan over medium-low heat, toast the coconut for 1–2 minutes, stirring constantly, until golden brown. Coconut burns easily, so remove from heat immediately after cooking.
- Mash the squash and coconut milk together with a fork or handheld blender. Season with salt and pepper if desired, and top with toasted coconut.

Garlic Thyme Sweet Potato Oven Fries

Delicious and very filling.

Time: 5 minutes active; 35 minutes to cook • Makes 2 servings

2 medium sweet potatoes
2 cloves garlic
2 tbsp coarsely chopped pumpkin seeds
1 tbsp thyme

1 ½ tbsp coconut oil
½ tbsp basil
Sea salt to taste

- Preheat oven to 300°F.
- Cut the sweet potatoes into wedges or chunks. In bowl, combine the garlic, pumpkin seeds, thyme, coconut oil, basil, and sea salt.
- Add the sweet potatoes, stirring with your hands to make sure all the pieces are covered with the mixture.
- Spread the sweet potatoes on a baking tray lightly oiled with coconut oil; bake for about 35 minutes.
- If you prefer the potatoes crispier, leave in the oven for an extra 5–10 minutes.

Kitchari

JIVAMUKTEA CAFÉ, MANHATTAN, NEW YORK

This is based on a traditional Indian porridge-like dish. It is very grounding and stabilizing without being too filling. It is often used in Ayurveda as a detox fast.

Time: 2 minutes active; 1 hour to cook • Makes 4 servings

2 cups red lentils

1 cup short-grain brown rice or white
   basmati rice

8 cups water

1 tbsp salt

- Place the lentils and rice in a large soup pot; wash and rinse with cold water 3 times.
- Add the water and bring to boil.
- Boil for 5 minutes, then turn heat to medium-low and cook for 1 hour.
- Add salt, stir well, and serve.

Spirulina Green Millet

JIVAMUKTEA CAFÉ, MANHATTAN, NEW YORK

Offers carbohydrate and chlorophyll-rich simplicity.

Time: 15 minutes active; 20 minutes to cook • Makes 1 serving

1 cup dry millet

2 cups water

4 tbsp flaxseed oil

4 tbsp powdered spirulina

1 tbsp Braggs Liquid Aminos
   (or soy sauce)

- Boil the millet in the water, reduce heat, and cook until all water is absorbed (about 20 minutes).
- Wait for the millet to "dry out" (about 10 minutes).
- Transfer the millet to large bowl. Add the oil and, using a large fork, mix well.
- Sprinkle spirulina over the millet and continue to mix well.
- Finally, add Braggs, mixing well until the millet is bright green.

Red Lentil Dal

THE GREEN DOOR, OTTAWA, ONTARIO

The Indian classic.

Time: 10 minutes, 30–45 minutes to cook • Makes 8–10 servings

2 cups red lentils
5 cups water
2 tbsp olive oil
1 tsp whole cumin seeds
¼ tsp asafetida (hing)
½ tsp garam masala
½ tsp ground cumin
¼ tsp ground cardamom
¼ tsp cayenne or 1 hot pepper, diced
2 cloves garlic, crushed
1 tsp salt, or to taste
¼ cup chopped fresh cilantro, for garnish
1 small tomato, diced, for garnish

- Wash the lentils well by rinsing and pouring off 3 changes of water. Cook the lentils in the water until well done (30–45 minutes). Do not drain. Set aside.
- Put a medium-sized pot on low heat. Add the oil and whole cumin seeds. Fry until they smell toasted.
- Add the rest of the spices and cayenne or hot pepper, and toast lightly. Add the garlic and sauté until light brown.
- Add the red lentils and salt. Cook on low heat for 10 minutes. Garnish with chopped cilantro and tomato.
- This will make a fairly thick dal. Add water for a thinner consistency.

Grilled Spinach with Salsa Rustica
(Italian Tomato Relish)

HORIZONS, PHILADELPHIA, PENNSYLVANIA

Bursting with flavor.

Time: 15 minutes • Makes 4 servings

SPINACH

2 tbsp olive oil
1 tsp minced garlic
1 pound washed baby spinach
Salt and pepper

- In a large skillet, heat the olive oil and garlic and toss the spinach until just past half-cooked.
- Season with salt and pepper.

SALSA

1 cup diced plum tomatoes
1 tsp capers
1 tsp chopped black olives
1 tsp chopped fresh oregano or thyme or both
2 tsp minced red onion
1 tsp olive oil
½ tsp sherry vinegar
Pinch of salt
¼ tsp black pepper

- Toss all of the salsa ingredients together and serve over the spinach.

Raw

Tabouli

GORILLA FOOD, VANCOUVER, BRITISH COLUMBIA

A raw twist on a classic.

Time: 10 minutes • Makes 2 servings

2–3 medium tomatoes, diced
⅓ medium cucumber, seeded and diced
10 sprigs parsley
1 tbsp lemon juice
¼ tsp salt
1 tbsp olive oil

- Mix the diced tomatoes and cucumbers. With a knife, hand-mince parsley and stir into the cucumber and tomato mix.
- Add the lemon juice, salt, and olive oil and mix well.

Raw

Couscous Flower

CRUDESSENCE, MONTREAL, QUEBEC

Raw, fiber-rich, and delicious.

Time: 5 minutes • Makes 8 servings

8 cups cauliflower, shredded in food processor
3 ½ ounces zucchini, diced
1 ounce onions, finely sliced
3 ½ ounces parsley, chopped
5 ounces tomatoes, diced
½ cup currants

3 tbsp lemon juice
3 tbsp olive oil
1 tsp sea salt
¼ tsp garlic purée
3 tbsp cumin
¼ tsp ground black pepper

- Mix all ingredients together by hand in a large salad bowl.

Almond Cakes with Mango Tartar Sauce

LIVE ORGANIC FOOD BAR, TORONTO, ONTARIO

Raw

Flavorful and filling, these cakes may be served as a side or a complete meal.

Time: 40 minutes; 12–18 hours to soak and dehydrate
Makes 6 servings (about 24 cakes and 2½ cups of sauce)

ALMOND CAKES

¼ bunch of celery

2 cups + 1 tbsp of soaked almonds

1 tbsp olive oil

Juice of 3 ½ limes

Water to blend

¼ cup of dulse flakes

2–3 green onions, thinly sliced with some green + some for garnish

1 ¼ inch of ginger, grated

⅛ cup of Nama Shoyu soy sauce

Celtic sea salt if needed

Fresh dill, for garnish

- In a food processor, start by pulsing the celery into pulp. Place in a medium-size mixing bowl. Set aside.
- In the food processor, add the almonds, olive oil, lime juice, and as much water as needed to blend into a fine, smooth mixture. Add this blended mixture to the bowl with the celery. Mix in remaining ingredients by hand. Season with Celtic sea salt if needed.
- Take 2 tbsp of dough and form into croquette shapes (mini patties) and dehydrate for at least 12–18 hours at 115°F until crisp on outside but moist in the middle.

MANGO TARTAR SAUCE

½ mango, peeled, pitted, and diced

¼ piece of red onion, diced

¼ English cucumbers, diced

½ daikon radish, peeled and diced

1 tbsp capers

2 tbsp chopped dill

½ tbsp rice wine vinegar

1 tbsp agave nectar

- In a medium mixing bowl, mix all ingredients. Chill for at least 30 minutes in a refrigerator before serving. This mix will last for at least 3–4 days in a refrigerator.

To serve
- Top each Almond Cake with 1 tsp Mango Tartar Sauce. Garnish with additional green onions and fresh dill.

Bok Choy Couscous with Sacha Inchi

Toasting the millet helps give it better texture and flavor.

Time: 10 minutes prep; 30 minutes to cook • Makes 2 servings

¾ cups dry millet
2 cups water
1 tbsp miso paste
1 tbsp sesame oil
2 tsp brown rice vinegar
½ tsp ume plum vinegar
1 tbsp minced shallot
2 cloves garlic, minced
2 tsp peeled and grated ginger
1 ½ pounds baby bok choy, leaves separated from the stems
2 tbsp yacon syrup
⅓ cup coarsely chopped sacha inchi

- Toast the millet in a frying pan over medium high heat for 3–4 minutes, or until the millet is fragrant and begins to sound as if it is popping.
- In a medium saucepan, combine the water, toasted millet, and miso paste. Bring to a boil, then reduce heat to a simmer.
- Cook uncovered until the water is absorbed (about 30 minutes), let stand for 5 minutes, then fluff with a fork.
- Once the millet has finished cooking, prepare the vegetables. Heat the sesame oil over medium-high heat. Add the shallot and garlic, and cook for 30 seconds until slightly carmelized. Add the baby bok choy and the prepared ginger–yacon mixture. Toss to combine. Cover and cook for 3–5 minutes, or until the bok choy is bright green and tender crisp (add a little water to the pan to prevent burning, if needed).
- Remove from heat. Place the millet in a large serving bowl and top with the contents of the cooked vegetable pan. Mix well. Sprinkle the sacha inchi seeds on top and serve warm.

Rustic Sweet Onion Flatbread

Satisfying like bread but light and with intense flavor. If you like you can use a dehydrator for this recipe instead of the oven.

Time: 10 minutes active; cooking time varies • Makes 8 servings

¾ cup tomato, chopped

⅓ cup raisins

1 tbsp miso paste

1 red onion, chopped (about 2 cups)

1 large garlic clove, chopped

¾ cup flaxseed powder

½ cup hemp seeds

2 tbsp chia seeds

- Preheat the oven to 250°F and line a baking sheet with parchment paper.
- In a food processor, blend the tomato, raisins, and miso paste together until smooth.
- Add the onion, garlic, and flaxseed powder and blend again as smooth as possible. Mix in the hemp seeds and chia seeds by hand.

Dehydrator method (preferred)
- Spread the mixture onto several teflex sheets, and dehydrate at desired temperature until dried out into a flatbread. For best results, flip over after 8–10 hours to allow even dehydration.

Oven method
- Pour the mixture onto the lined baking sheet. Use a spatula to spread into a thin layer, forming about a 10 × 14-inch rectangle (spread as evenly as possible to ensure even cooking).
- Bake for 1 hour, then remove from oven and place another sheet of parchment paper on top of the spread. Holding the two layers together, flip the whole spread over so that the new parchment is on the bottom. Carefully peel away the top layer of parchment from the spread and discard.
- Return to the oven for 15–20 minutes, or until the edges begin to brown slightly. Turn off the oven, and leave the tray inside until the oven has cooled, about 30 minutes. Break into larger pieces for flatbread, into smaller pieces for crackers, or crumble into croutons.

Roasted Garlic Quinoa

One of the healthiest and tastiest ways to infuse quinoa with flavor.

Time: 5 minutes; 30 minutes to cook • Makes 3–4 servings

1 whole head garlic, roasted
2 tbsp melted coconut oil + some for drizzling
1 tsp lemon juice
4 cups cooked quinoa
½ tsp sea salt, or to taste
½ tsp fresh thyme leaves, for garnish

- To roast the garlic, heat the oven to 400°F. Cut off the top of the head of garlic, about ¼–½ inch down, and place it inside a small piece of aluminum foil.
- Drizzle with coconut oil, close the foil loosely, and bake for 30 minutes. Open foil after removing from the oven.
- Once the garlic has cooled, squeeze the roasted garlic cloves out of the peel and into a small bowl.
- Add the coconut oil and lemon juice and mix well. Pour the resulting sauce into a medium saucepan and heat on medium-low heat.
- Add the quinoa and sea salt and cook, stirring, for 2–3 minutes until quinoa is heated through and the flavors have incorporated. Garnish with fresh thyme before serving.

Superfood Gomashio

Sprinkle on top of salads, rice, and quinoa for a flavorful salty condiment. You can also skip the toasting step and use raw.

Time: 5 minutes • Makes ⅔ cup

4 sheets nori
¼ cup hemp seeds
¼ cup sesame seeds

1 tsp sea salt
1 tsp sesame oil

- Rip or crumble the nori into small flakes over a bowl. Slowly spoon into a running food processor.
- Add the hemp seeds, a little at a time, stopping the machine if needed to scrape down the sides and re-incorporate ingredients. Add the sesame seeds, sea salt, and sesame oil.
- Heat a small frying pan over medium heat. Add the mixture, and toast for about 1 minute, stirring constantly, just until the nori is crisp and fragrant and begins to shrink in size.
- Remove from heat quickly to prevent burning. This will keep for several weeks in an airtight container.

Baby Zucchini and Avocado Tartar

MATTHEW KENNEY

This recipe calls for ring molds.

Time: 10 minutes • Serves 4

2 firm avocados, finely diced
4–5 baby zucchini, finely diced
2 tbsp lemon juice
1 tbsp olive oil + drizzle, for garnish
2 tbsp micro basil (or finely minced basil)

1 tbsp chives, minced + some
  for garnish
1 tsp agave
2–3 tsp coarse salt
Freshly ground pepper, for garnish

- Toss all ingredients until well combined.
- To serve, divide into four servings and press into ring molds. Garnish with chive, freshly ground pepper, and a drizzle of olive oil.

Simple Italian Zucchini Noodles

A classic example of the Italian mastery of letting beautiful ingredients shine.

Time: 15 minutes active prep • Makes 4 servings

4 medium yellow zucchini
1 tsp sea salt
1 tbsp coconut oil
5 large cloves garlic, minced
2 tbsp hemp oil
¼ tsp red pepper flakes

- Trim the ends of the zucchini. Using a hand-held vegetable peeler, carefully strip the zucchini, layer by layer, into noodle-like pieces and gather into a colander (for best results, discard the watery center section that holds the seeds).
- Toss the zucchini strips with the sea salt, then place the colander over a large bowl to catch excess moisture. Leave the zucchini to rest for 30 minutes.
- After 30 minutes, wash the zucchini thoroughly with warm water to remove any excess salt and let drain for 5 more minutes.
- Heat the coconut oil over medium heat, and add the garlic. Cook for 1–2 minutes until the garlic begins to turn golden.
- Add the zucchini and toss well, cooking for 1 minute longer or until heated through.
- Remove from heat and toss with hemp oil and red pepper flakes, adding more sea salt to taste. Serve warm.

Almond Noodles with Carrots and Wakame

This recipe takes noodles with peanut sauce to the next level.

Time: 20 minutes • Makes 4 servings

NOODLES

2 packages kelp noodles (24 ounces)
3 tbsp almond butter
1½ tbsp yacon syrup
1 tbsp brown rice miso
1 tsp wasabi powder
¼ tsp garlic powder
1 tsp ginger powder
¼ cup water, or more as needed
1 tsp sesame oil
2 medium carrots, grated

GARNISH

1 scallion, sliced thin (white and green parts)
2 tbsp almonds, chopped

- Rinse the kelp noodles thoroughly and place in a pot of warm water. Let soak for 10 minutes to soften.
- While the noodles are soaking, whisk the almond butter, yacon syrup, miso, wasabi, garlic, ginger, and water in a bowl or blender until smooth. Set aside.
- Gently heat the sesame oil over medium heat in a large frying pan or wok. Add the kelp noodles and carrots and stir fry for 2–3 minutes, tossing to ensure even cooking. Add the almond sauce and cook for 2 more minutes, or until the sauce has thickened.
- Transfer to a serving bowl and top with scallions and chopped almonds.

Variation: This may also be served as a raw dish. Simply reduce the amount of water in the sauce to 1–2 tbsp, and omit the sesame oil entirely. Instead of cooking, just toss the ingredients together and serve at room temperature.

Roasted Broccoli with Avocado Pesto

Fiber and flavor rich—delicious.

Time: 20 minutes • Makes 4 servings

BROCCOLI

3 pounds broccoli, cut into florets (including some stem)
2 tbsp melted coconut oil
Salt and freshly ground pepper

SAUCE

1 medium avocado
4 cloves garlic
3 packed cups fresh parsley leaves + 2 tbsp for garnish
¼ cup lemon juice
2 heaping tbsp packed dulse
½ tsp sea salt

- Preheat the oven to 475°F. Line a baking sheet with aluminum foil for easy clean-up.
- Toss the broccoli with the coconut oil and sprinkle with salt and pepper. Spread out on the baking sheet and roast for 15 minutes or until tender-crisp, tossing the broccoli halfway through.
- While the broccoli is cooking, make the sauce. Mash the avocado in a small bowl and place in a food processor. With the machine running, add the garlic, parsley, lemon juice, dulse, and sea salt and process until a smooth paste has formed.
- Toss the avocado mixture with the hot broccoli in a large bowl, then transfer to a serving plate and sprinkle with reserved 2 tbsp parsley.

Fresh Pasta Puttanesca

A vegetable-in-place-of-pasta twist on a classic.

Time: 15 minutes prep; 1 hour to soak and sit • Makes 4 servings

PASTA

4 large zucchini
1 ½ tbsp Vega Antioxidant EFA Oil Blend (or use hemp oil or virgin olive oil)
Pinch of sea salt

SAUCE

4 sun-dried tomatoes
1 ½ cups cherry tomatoes, quartered
1 tsp pressed garlic
4 tsp dulse flakes
3 tbsp Vega Antioxidant & EFA Oil Blend (or use hemp oil or flaxseed oil)
½ cup kalamata olives, pitted
¼ cup fresh parsley, chopped
½ tsp red pepper flakes
¼ tsp sea salt

- To begin the sauce, place the sun-dried tomatoes in enough water to cover them. Set aside and let soak for 45 minutes or until soft.
- To make the "pasta," use a vegetable peeler to dispose of green skin on the zucchini, then peel long fettuccini-like strips with the rest. Toss strips in the oil and sea salt until well coated, and set aside for 15 minutes to soften.
- To make the sauce, put sun-dried tomatoes (once soaking is complete) along with the remaining sauce ingredients into a food processor. Pulse until just finely chopped, about 5 or 6 times.
- Toss sauce with pasta and serve, sprinkling with extra parsley if desired.
- The sauce also works as a cooked recipe. Simmer on low heat for 3–4 minutes until just heated through, and then serve with the pasta.

Optional: If you have a dehydrator and a little patience, spread sauce on a teflex sheet before mixing with pasta, and dehydrate for an hour—deliciousness will result. Stir before combining with pasta, and serve warm.

Cheesy Broccoli Bowl

I like to serve this recipe as is (uncooked), enjoying the maximum nutritional potential of these great superfoods. If you're craving a warm dish though, no worries—simply steam the florets lightly for a few minutes, then combine with the sauce. Either way, the delicious cheesy flavor and addictive broccoli crunch will have you coming back for a healthy second round every time.

Time: 10 minutes • Makes 4 servings

2 tbsp nutritional yeast
½ tsp paprika
¼ tsp garlic powder
¼ cup raw tahini
1 tsp brown rice or chickpea miso paste
3 tsp lemon juice
2 tbsp coconut oil, melted
3 tbsp water, if needed
1 ½ tsp ume plum vinegar
8 cups finely chopped fresh broccoli florets
2–3 tbsp hemp seeds

- In a small bowl, mix the nutritional yeast, paprika, and garlic powder together. Stir in the tahini and brown rice or chickpea miso paste.
- Pour in the lemon juice, coconut oil, water, and ume plum vinegar, and whisk thoroughly. If a thinner sauce is desired, add extra water, a tablespoon at a time.
- Put the broccoli into a larger bowl and pour sauce on top. Toss until evenly coated (for best results, use your hands!).
- Sprinkle with hemp seeds and serve.
- Keeps refrigerated for several days.

spreads, dips, sauces, and dressings

Traditionally, spreads are spread on bread. But in sticking with my dietary philosophy, I use them mostly on raw vegetables.

Zucchini Hummus

GORILLA FOOD, VANCOUVER, BRITISH COLUMBIA

A lighter version than the traditional chickpea hummus, with zucchini as its base.

Time: 5 minutes • Makes 1 ½ cups

1 cup sesame seeds
2–3 medium cloves garlic
10 sprigs parsley
5 tbsp lemon juice
⅓ tsp salt
3 medium zucchini, cut into 1-inch pieces

- Grind the sesame seeds with the S-blade in a dry food processor until it is a creamy tahini. Set this paste aside in a bowl.
- Finely mince the garlic with the S-blade in the food processor.
- Add parsley, lemon juice, salt, and zucchini and blend until nearly puréed.
- Add the tahini back in and blend all ingredients together until smooth and creamy.

Zucky Hummus

CRUDESSENCE, MONTREAL, QUEBEC

With sunflower seeds and zucchini as its base, this hummus's flavor is further enhanced by the ginger.

Time: 10 minutes active; 8 hours presoak • Makes 4 ½ cups

1 ½ cups of sunflower seeds (soaked for 8 hours)
2 ¼ cups coarsely chopped zucchini
¼ cup lemon juice
¼ cup water
¼ cup olive oil
1 tsp ginger juice
1 tsp sea salt
2 tsp cumin
3 cloves garlic
Pinch cayenne powder

- Soak the sunflower seeds for 8 hours.
- Rinse the soaked seeds well before use. Mix all ingredients together in a blender until creamy and smooth.

Pecan and Dill Pâté

CRUDESSENCE, MONTREAL, QUEBEC

You can use this pâté to replace the rice in sushi rolls. Just make them as usual, with a lot of finely chopped veggies and avocado to replace the fish … simply amazing!

Time: 10 minutes active; 8 hours presoak • Makes 6 cups

3 cups sunflower seeds (soaked for 8 hours)
2 cups pecans
¼ cup apple cider vinegar
¼ cup lemon juice
½ cup sunflower oil
¼ cup water
1 cup fresh parsley, chopped coarsely (packed firmly)
½ cup fresh dill chopped coarsely (packed firmly)
3 cloves garlic
2 tsp sea salt

- Soak the sunflower seeds for 8 hours.
- Rinse the soaked seeds well before use. Using a food processor, grind them into a powder.
- Add the rest of the ingredients and mix until a creamy texture without lumps is obtained.

Walnut Chili Pâté

GORILLA FOOD, VANCOUVER, BRITISH COLUMBIA

Filling, yet easy to digest and packed with vegetables, this pâté has an intense flavor.

Time: 10 minutes active, 6–8 hours presoak • Makes 1 cup

½ cup sunflower seeds (soaked overnight)
⅓ cup walnuts (soaked overnight)
2 stalks celery
¼ medium zucchini
¼ bunch cilantro
5 sprigs parsley
½ tbsp lemon juice
¼ tsp salt
¹⁄₁₆ tsp cayenne chili powder
¼ tsp chili blend powder
¹⁄₁₆ tsp cumin
¹⁄₁₆ tsp coriander

- Soak the seeds and nuts for 6–8 hours or overnight and rinse well before using.
- In a food processor with the S-blade, coarse-grind the sunflower seeds and walnuts. Put in a medium-size bowl.
- With the food processor and the S-blade, purée celery, zucchini, cilantro, parsley, lemon juice, salt, cayenne chili powder, chili blend powder, cumin, and coriander.
- Add this purée into the seed and nut mix and mix everything well by hand.

Sacha Inchi Sunflower Seed Pâté

This mild pâté is a great accompaniment to flavored crackers.

Time: 10 minutes • Makes about 2 cups

2 cloves garlic
1 cup sacha inchi seeds
1 cup sunflower seeds
½ cup walnuts

⅓ cup hemp oil
¼ cup orange juice
1 tsp sea salt

- In a food processor, process all ingredients together until smooth. Keep refrigerated for up to 2 weeks.

Creamy Cilantro Tahini Pâté

BLOSSOMING LOTUS, PORTLAND, OREGON

Smooth and flavorful, this pâté is ideal for vegetable dipping or to add to a salad for a nutritional boost.

Time: 15 minutes active; 2 hours presoak • Makes about 4 servings

2 cups sunflower seeds (soaked 2 hours)
2 cups rough chopped fresh cilantro
1 ½ peeled garlic cloves
1 ½ tbsp chopped jalapeño
3 tbsp small diced yellow onion
6 tbsp fresh lemon juice

2 tsp agave
6 tbsp raw tahini
3 tbsp olive oil
1 ½ tbsp ground cumin
1 tsp salt

- Soak the sunflower seeds for 2 hours, rinse, and drain.
- Clean the cilantro and chop thoroughly.
- Blend everything except sunflower seeds in a blender, put into large container, add sunflower seeds, and stir. Blend in batches in food processor. Adjust salt to taste.

Sacha Inchi Butter

A delicious omega-3-rich, nut-free alternative to peanut butter.

Time: 10 minutes • Makes ¾ cup

1 cup sacha inchi seeds
2 tsp hemp oil
Dash of sea salt

- Using a food processor quipped with the S-blade, process all ingredients for 5–10 minutes, or until desired creaminess is reached. Remove with rubber spatula.

Sacha Inchi and Sunflower Seed Chocolate Spread

A delicious, healthy, omega-3-rich, nut-free alternative to Nutella.

Time: 10 minutes active; 8 hours presoak

½ cup sacha inchi seeds
1 cup sunflower seeds
2 tbsp roasted carob powder
1 large pitted date (fresh or soaked for 8 hours)

- Using a food processor quipped with the S-blade, process all ingredients for 5–10 minutes, or until desired creaminess is reached. Remove with rubber spatula.

Seasonal Fig Jam

Great on toasted sprouted bread, or atop a warm morning porridge. The riper/softer the figs, the sweeter the jam. Make when figs are at their peak ripeness.

Time: 5 minutes • Makes about 1 cup

1 cup chopped fresh, very ripe figs (such as black mission)
3–4 large Medjool dates, pits removed (amount depends on
    how naturally sweet the figs are)
1 tbsp lemon juice
⅓ cup apple juice
2 tbsp chia seeds

- Place all ingredients in a blender and process until smooth.
- Cover and refrigerate mixture for 30 minutes before serving to allow the chia seeds to thicken the mixture. It will keep for 3–4 days, refrigerated.

Fresh Fruit Strawberry Jam

Excellent on crispy crackers or as a dessert spread/sauce.

Time: 10 minutes active; 30 minutes to chill • Makes about 1 cup

1 ½ cup diced strawberries
3 large Medjool dates, pits removed
1 tbsp lemon juice
1 tbsp chia seeds

- Use a blender to blend *half* of the strawberries with the dates, lemon juice, and chia seeds until smooth.
- Stop machine and add the remaining strawberries. Pulse blender several times until berries are incorporated yet still chunky.
- Cover and refrigerate mixture for 30 minutes before serving to allow the chia seeds to thicken the jam and the flavors to develop. It will keep for 3–4 days, refrigerated.

Guacamole

GORILLA FOOD, VANCOUVER, BRITISH COLUMBIA

Classic, simple guacamole.

Time: 10 minutes • Makes 1 cup

2 medium avocados
1 ½ tbsp lemon juice
½ tsp salt
⅛ small onion

- Mash the avocado, lemon juice, and salt together with a fork. With a knife, finely mince the onion and mix into the avocado mash-up.

Ranch Dipping Sauce

Serve as a dip for homemade root fries or carrots, or even as a salad dressing.

Time: 10 minutes • Makes about 1 cup

1 cup young coconut meat (about 2 coconuts)
⅓ cup young coconut water (add additional if needed for blending)
2 tbsp apple cider vinegar
1 ¼ tsp onion powder
½ tsp sea salt
¼ tsp dried dill
1 medium clove garlic

- Use a blender to blend all ingredients together until creamy and smooth. Add additional coconut water if needed to blend properly.

Lemon Tahini Dipping Sauce

Ideal with carrots, celery, and cucumber.

Time: 5 minutes • Makes about ½ cup

3 tbsp tahini
3 tbsp lemon juice
3 tbsp water
¼ tsp garlic powder
1 minced scallion (white and light green parts only)
1 tbsp minced parsley

- Mix all the ingredients together in a jar. Refrigerate when not in use—it will keep for several weeks.

Salsa

GORILLA FOOD, VANCOUVER, BRITISH COLUMBIA

Flavorful fresh raw salsa can be added to a salad or can be eaten simply with an avocado.

Time: 10 minutes • Makes about 1 cup

1 fresh date
⅛ tsp sea salt
1/16 tsp cayenne chilies
1 tbsp lemon juice

⅛ medium yellow onion
2 medium tomatoes
¼ bunch cilantro

- In a food processor with the S-blade, blend the date, salt, and cayenne chilies. Slowly add the lemon juice to blend the dates until fully clear.
- Add the onions and tomatoes to the food processor and pulse-chop everything into a saucy but still chunky consistency. Pour into a bowl.
- With a knife, hand-mince the cilantro and stir well into the mix.

Sacha Inchi Black Bean Lime Salsa

Protein, micronutrient, and EFA rich, this salsa is a nutritional powerhouse.

Time: 10 minutes active; 2–3 hours to soak • Makes about 2 cups

Juice of ½ lime
2 cloves garlic, finely chopped
1 tomato, diced
½ onion, diced
1 cup black beans
1 cup coarsely chopped or torn cilantro

1 tbsp balsamic vinegar
1 tbsp hemp oil
½ cup chopped sacha inchi seeds
½ tsp cayenne pepper
¼ tsp sea salt

- In a bowl, combine all ingredients. Allow the salsa to sit for a few hours at room temperature so that the flavors infuse.
- Keep refrigerated for up to 1 week.

Hemp Black-Eyed Pea Cayenne Salsa

This is an ideal salsa to add protein-packed spicy flavor to your vegetables.

Time: 10 minutes active; 2–3 hours to sit • Makes about 2 cups

Juice of 1 lemon
1 tomato, diced
½ onion, diced
1 cup black-eyed peas
1 cup coarsely chopped or torn cilantro
1 tbsp balsamic vinegar

1 tbsp hemp oil
2 tbsp hemp seeds
½ tsp cayenne pepper
½ tsp chili flakes
¼ tsp sea salt

- In a bowl, combine all ingredients. Allow the mixture to sit for a few hours at room temperature so that the flavors infuse.
- Keep refrigerated, for up to 1 week.

Yellow Bell Pepper Pine Cheese

LIFE FOOD GOURMET, MIAMI, FLORIDA

Flavor-packed and full of nutrition, thanks to the nutritional yeast.

Time: 5 minutes • Makes 1 cup

1 yellow bell pepper
½ cup pine nuts
3 ½ tbsp nutritional yeast
1 tsp sea salt
1 tsp tarragon

1 tbsp olive oil
1 tsp apple cider vinegar
1 tsp agave nectar
1 small clove garlic

- Place all ingredients in a Vita-Mix or regular blender and blend thoroughly.

Live Cashew Cheese Base

BLOSSOMING LOTUS, PORTLAND, OREGON

Ideal as a base for other recipes or any time you need a cheese-like substitute. The rejuvelac (a liquid made from fermented grains) is rich in healthy bacteria that aid in digestion.

Time: 5 minutes active; 8 hours to sit • Makes about 2 ½ cups

2 cups soaked cashews
¾ cup rejuvelac

- Soak cashews overnight. Then rinse well, drain, and blend cashews in food processor. Slowly add the rejuvelac until the mixture is thick and creamy.
- Let the mixture sit at room temperature overnight to ferment. Don't fully cover, so that gases can escape.
- Refrigerate when fermenting time is over.

Live Seasoned Cashew Cheese

BLOSSOMING LOTUS, PORTLAND, OREGON

Ideal as a topping for steamed broccoli, cauliflower, and carrots.

Time: 5 minutes (once Live Cashew Cheese Base is made)
Makes about 5 servings

2 ½ cups Live Cashew Cheese Base (see p. 204)
Pinch sea salt
Pinch black pepper
1 tsp extra-virgin olive oil (can substitute hemp oil)

- Put all ingredients into a blender. Blend until smooth.

Live Cashew Sour Cream

BLOSSOMING LOTUS, PORTLAND, OREGON

"Live," in that it's made with soaked (germinated) nuts, this recipe is creamy yet easy to digest.

Time: 5 minutes (once Live Seasoned Cashew Cheese is made)
Makes about 10 servings

1 ¼ cups Live Seasoned Cashew Cheese (see above)
4 tsp fresh lemon juice
½ tsp sea salt
Pinch black pepper
4 tsp extra-virgin olive oil (can be substituted with hemp oil)
2 ½ tbsp filtered water

- Blend all ingredients in food processor.

Marinara/Pizza Sauce

Light and flavorful, this is a versatile sauce.

Time: 5 minutes active; 15 minutes to soak • Makes 4 cups

1 ½ sun-dried tomatoes

2 Roma tomatoes

¼ cup olive oil

1 ½ tbsp Italian seasoning

1 tbsp oregano

1 handful fresh basil

2 tbsp palm nectar granuals

1 tsp apple cider vinegar

1 ½ tsp sun-dried sea salt

1 tbsp anise seeds (optional)

- Soak sun-dried tomatoes for about 15 minutes. Blend all ingredients except sun-dried tomatoes. Add sun-dried tomatoes and blend again.

UnMotza Macadamia Cheese Sauce

For a lighter recipe, substitute the macadamia nuts with pumpkin seeds. Always use a rubber spatula to scrape the sides of the processor and get an even mixture.

Time: 5 minutes • Makes about 3 cups

1 ½ cups macadamia nuts

1 ½ cups Irish moss gel

½ cups nutritional yeast

2 tsp sun-dried sea salt

¼ cup nut milk

- Place nuts in a food processor with an S-blade and grind them into a thick paste. Add the remaining ingredients and pulse a few more times.

Sun-Dried Tomato Sauce

CRUDESSENCE, MONTREAL, QUEBEC

This flavor-packed versatile sauce can be used on pizzas or as a tasty accompaniment for roasted vegetables.

Time: 10 minutes • Makes about 5 cups

2 ½ cups sun-dried tomatoes
5 medium fresh tomatoes, quartered
1 carrot, sliced coarsely
1 tbsp garlic paste
1 tbsp olive oil
½ cup Mediterranean spices
½ tsp cayenne powder
½ cup onion, sliced coarsely
½ cup onion, finely sliced
½ cup parsley, finely chopped

- Rehydrate the sun-dried tomatoes in a bowl of water while you gather the other ingredients.
- In the blender, process the rehydrated tomatoes (without the soaking water) with the rest of the ingredients except the onions and parsley.
- Do not fill the blender more than ⅔ full at a time. You may have to repeat the process a few times, placing the fresh tomatoes in the bottom of the blender and adding the other ingredients on top.
- Pour the tomato mixture into a bowl, and fold in the coarsely sliced and finely chopped onions and the chopped parsley.

Note: Mediterranean spices can be bought as a mix. The spices include annatto, cumin, oregano, sweet and hot paprikas, rosemary, and saffron.

Live Avocado Goddess Sauce

BLOSSOMING LOTUS, PORTLAND, OREGON

Can be used as a chip or vegetable dip, or as an addition to a salad.

Time: 15 minutes • Makes about 3 cups

2 ripe avocados
2 ½ tbsp apple cider vinegar
2 tsp minced garlic
1 tbsp red onion
½ tbsp dried parsley
½ tsp salt

2 tsp ground cumin
½ tsp pepper
1 ½ tbsp nutritional yeast
2 ½ tbsp fresh lemon juice
1 cup filtered water

- Put all ingredients in a large container and blend with an immersion wand until smooth with a medium thickness. Add more salt, apple cider vinegar, and lemon juice to taste.
- Store in the refrigerator for up to 10 days.

Cashew–Truffle Oil Cream

MILLENNIUM RESTAURANT, SAN FRANCISCO, CALIFORNIA

Tastes as fancy as it sounds.

Time: 10 minutes active; 1 hour presoak

4 tbsp raw cashews, presoaked in warm
  water 1 hour
2 tsp nutritional yeast
Water as needed

1 tsp balsamic vinegar
Black truffle oil to taste
Salt to taste

- Rinse and drain the cashews. In a blender, blend the cashews with the yeast and enough water to just cover the nuts.
- Slowly add more water while blending until the consistency is that of thickened cream.
- Add the balsamic vinegar, truffle oil, and salt to taste.

Regular, Thick, and Whipped Cashew Cream

Tal Ronnen

To make the regular cashew cream into thick cream, reduce the amount of water in the blender so that the water just covers the cashews.

Time: 10 minutes active; overnight presoak
Makes about 3 ½ cups regular cream or 2 ¼ cups thick cream

2 cups whole raw cashews (not pieces, which are often dry), rinsed very well
    under cold water

- Put the cashews in a bowl and add cold water to cover them. Cover the bowl and refrigerate overnight.
- Drain the cashews and rinse under cold water. Place in a blender with enough fresh cold water to cover them by 1 inch.
- Blend on high for several minutes until very smooth. (If you're not using a professional high-speed blender, such as a Vita-Mix, which creates an ultra-smooth cream, strain the cashew cream through a fine-mesh sieve.)

WHIPPED VARIATION

Lighter and possibly more delicious than cashew cream.

Time: 5 minutes active (once Thick Cashew Cream is made); 2 hours to chill
Makes about 2 cups

1 cup Thick Cashew Cream (see above) ¼ cup water
¼ cup light agave nectar ⅔ cup refined coconut oil, warmed
½ tsp vanilla extract   until liquid

- Place the Thick Cashew Cream in a blender and add the agave nectar, vanilla, and ¼ cup water. Blend until thoroughly combined.
- With the blender running, slowly drizzle the liquid coconut oil in through the hole in the blender lid. Blend until emulsified.
- Pour into a bowl and chill in the refrigerator, covered, for 2 hours. Stir before serving.

Spiced Sesame Sauce

GORILLA FOOD, VANCOUVER, BRITISH COLUMBIA

Ideal on raw, steamed, or stir-fried vegetables.

Time: 10 minutes • Makes 1 cup

⅓ cup sesame seeds
1 ½ tbsp lemon juice
⅔ cup water
⅛ tsp salt
½ tsp cumin

¼ tsp paprika
½ date
1/16 tsp cayenne
5 sprigs parsley

- In a blender, combine all ingredients except the parsley and blend until smooth. With a knife, mince the parsley and place in a bowl.
- Pour the sauce in with the parsley and stir together.

Miso Mushroom Gravy

LIVE ORGANIC FOOD BAR, TORONTO, ONTARIO

Great on your favorite nut loaf.

Time: 10 minutes • Makes about 4 cups

½ cup of olive oil
Juice of 1 lemon
3 stalks of celery, chopped
⅛ cup Nama Shoyu soy sauce

3 cloves garlic
1 ¾ cup miso (brown rice if possible)
¾ cup pitted dates
1 ¾ cup sliced button mushrooms

- In a blender, mix all ingredients except for the sliced mushrooms and blend until smooth.
- In a medium bowl, add the mushrooms to the gravy. This keeps for a few days in a cold refrigerator.

Roasted Garlic Dressing

CANDLE 79, MANHATTAN, NEW YORK

The chefs at Candle 79 say they always keep a good amount of Roasted Garlic Dressing on hand. Not only is it excellent on salads, but they also serve it with roasted or steamed vegetables, rice, and grains.

Time: 15 minutes active; 35–40 minutes to cook • Makes 2 cups

1 cup garlic cloves, peeled
1 cup extra-virgin olive oil
½ cup filtered water
¼ cup balsamic vinegar
¼ cup sherry wine vinegar or red wine vinegar
1 tbsp white miso
2 tbsp minced fresh thyme or 1 tsp dried oregano
Pinch of ground nutmeg
1 tsp sea salt
2 tsp freshly ground black pepper
¼ cup dried currants or cranberries (optional)

- Preheat oven to 350°F.
- Put the peeled garlic cloves in a baking dish and cover with extra-virgin olive oil. Cover the dish with foil and roast approximately 25 minutes or until golden brown. When cool enough to handle, remove the garlic with a slotted spoon and transfer to a blender.
- Reserve the roasted garlic oil for another use.
- Add the water, vinegars, miso, thyme or oregano, nutmeg, salt, and pepper to the garlic, and blend until smooth. Add a bit more water if necessary. Add currants or cranberries, if desired. The dressing will keep in the refrigerator, covered, for 1 week.

Note: The reserved roasted garlic oil will keep in a covered container for 1 week. Use it to drizzle over pasta, vegetables, and salad greens. It's also excellent when used in sautés and stir-fries.

Maple Cayenne Tahini Dressing

This is a full-flavored dressing with a bit of bite. The tahini offers a good amount of calcium, and the cayenne pepper helps get the blood flowing.

Time: 10 minutes • Makes about 1 ½ cups

½ clove garlic
½ cup balsamic vinegar
½ cup hemp oil
¼ cup water
2 tbsp tahini

½ tbsp dill
½ tsp cayenne pepper
¼ tsp maple syrup
Sea salt to taste

- Put all ingredients into a blender. Blend until smooth.

Garlic–Green Peppercorn Dressing

MILLENNIUM RESTAURANT, SAN FRANCISCO, CALIFORNIA

Smooth, with a bite of pepper, this dressing adds full-bodied flavor to any salad.

Time: 15 minutes • Makes 2 ½ cups

1 ½ cups Regular Cashew Cream
  (see p. 209)
1 tsp fine-ground green peppercorn
¼ tsp coarsely ground green peppercorn
¼ cup extra-virgin olive oil
Salt as needed

1 clove minced garlic
¼ cup cider vinegar
2 tsp nutritional yeast
1 tbsp minced fresh dill
1 tbsp minced fresh tarragon

- Blend the Regular Cashew Cream through the green peppercorn. Slowly emulsify in the oil.
- Adjust salt. Whisk in remaining ingredients.

Chili-Lime Dressing

BLOSSOMING LOTUS, PORTLAND, OREGON

A full-flavored, healthy version of the Mexican-inspired classic.

Time: 15 minutes • Makes about 10 servings

2 ½ peeled garlic cloves
1 tsp deseeded New Mexico pepper
Pinch cayenne pepper
2 tsp fresh orange juice
5 tbsp fresh lime juice
1 tbsp raw agave syrup
1 tsp cumin powder

2 tsp medium diced red onion
½ cup loosely packed fresh cilantro
½ avocado
½ cup filtered water
1 ½ tsp sea salt
12 tbsp olive oil or hemp oil

- In a blender, process the garlic, peppers, orange juice, and lime juice together until smooth.
- Add in the agave syrup, cumin, onion, and cilantro.
- Add the avocado, water, and salt. Blend and drizzle in oil while blender is on low.

Sweet Mustard Dressing

A twist on a traditional honey mustard dressing, this is ideal as a vegetable dip or salad dressing.

Time: 5 minutes • Makes about ⅔ cup

⅓ cup yacon syrup
¼ cup Dijon mustard
2 tbsp apple cider vinegar
4 tsp almond butter
½ tsp sea salt, or to taste

- Mix all ingredients together in a jar and keep refrigerated till ready to use.

Vinaigrette

Tal Ronnen

A simple classic.

Time: 5 minutes • Makes 2 servings

1 tbsp white wine vinegar
½ tsp agave nectar
3 tbsp extra-virgin olive oil
Sea salt and freshly ground black pepper

• Place the vinegar and agave nectar in a small bowl, then, whisking constantly, slowly pour in the oil in a thin stream. Season with salt and pepper to taste.

Lentil Dressing

Flavorful, protein-rich salad dressing.

Time: 5 minutes • Makes about ¾ cup

⅔ cup cooked green lentils, unsalted
6 tbsp olive oil
2 tsp miso paste
2 tsp Dijon mustard
4 tsp balsamic vinegar
Freshly cracked pepper

• Use a blender or food processor to blend the lentils, oil, miso, mustard, and vinegar into a semi-smooth mixture. Add pepper to taste.

Coconut-Cumin Dressing

Delicious creamy texture and a West Indian–inspired flavor. This dressing uses young Thai coconuts, which are white on the outside, unlike the more commonly found brown "hairy" ones, otherwise known as "old coconuts." Young Thai coconuts can be found in Whole Foods Markets and most health-food stores, as well as in Asian markets.

Time: 10 minutes • Makes about 1 cup

1 cup young coconut meat (about 2 coconuts)
2 tbsp young coconut water
1 ½ tbsp balsamic vinegar
2 tbsp lime juice
1 ¼ tsp cumin powder
1 medium clove garlic
2 tsp palm sugar
¼ tsp sea salt

• Blend all ingredients in a blender until smooth.

Creamy Thai Dressing

Matthew Kenney

Smooth, filling, and delicious, this is an ideal dressing for any salad.

Time: 10 minutes • Makes 2 ½ cups

¾ cup sesame oil
½ cup Nama Shoyu soy sauce
¼ cup olive oil
¼ cup lime juice

1 tbsp maple syrup
3 tsp red chili flakes
1 tsp sea salt
¼ cup chopped cashews

• Blend all ingredients in a blender until smooth.

Raw

Pasta with Marinara Sauce

KARYN'S FRESH CORNER CAFÉ, CHICAGO, ILLINOIS

Raw and light zucchini "pasta" with a fully-flavored sauce.

Time: 10 minutes prep; 30 minutes to marinate • Makes 4 servings

2 large zucchini
½ tbsp sea salt
¼ cup extra-virgin olive oil
1 ½ cups sun-dried tomatoes, soaked in water
4 cups fresh sweet tomatoes
2 cloves garlic
1 ½ tbsp agave nectar
¼ cup green olives
¼ cup black olives
1 cup basil
⅛ cup tamari

- Peel the zucchini (optional) and shred into long spaghetti strands with spiralizer or peeler.
- Marinate zucchini with the salt and 2 tbsp olive oil for 30 minutes.
- Gently squeeze out excess water.
- In a blender, process the sun-dried tomatoes with the soaking water, 2 cups of fresh tomatoes, garlic, and agave nectar. Pour in a large bowl.
- Slice or chop the olives, dice the remaining fresh tomatoes, chiffonade the basil and add them to bowl.
- Add the remaining olive oil and the tamari. Stir gently.
- Add drained zucchini to sauce and toss to coat.

Raw

Asian Noodle Bowl with Kelp Noodles and Almond Chili Sauce

CRU, LOS ANGELES, CALIFORNIA

A unique and filling sauce on light sea-vegetable noodles

Time: 10 minutes prep • Makes 2 servings

ALMOND CHILI SAUCE

½ cup raw almond butter
¼ cup tamari
¼ cup olive oil
⅛ cup lemon juice
⅛ cup water
¼ cup agave nectar
1 tsp salt
1 pinch chipotle powder
1 ½ tbsp chili flakes

- Mix everything together in a bowl until well combined.

NOODLES

½ cup shredded cabbage
1 cup kelp noodles
½ cup cucumbers, sliced

GARNISH

Cilantro, finely chopped
Radish sprouts
Cashews, chopped
Chilies, chopped

- Toss noodle ingredients with 1–2 ounces of the Almond Chili Sauce. Garnish with cilantro, radish sprouts, cashews, and chilies.

Pumpkin Gnocchi with Jerusalem Artichoke Purée

MILLENNIUM RESTAURANT, SAN FRANCISCO, CALIFORNIA

This is a wonderful dish. It is a bit more complex to make than some of the other recipes, but it's well worth the effort. You might want to first try this recipe on a weekend!

Prep time: 40 minutes • Makes 4 servings

GNOCCHI

2 large yellow Finn potatoes, baked
2 cups cooked pumpkin, skin removed
⅔ cup of all-purpose flour, plus more as needed
   (can use quinoa or buckwheat flour to make gluten free)
Salt to taste

- Remove the skin from potatoes. Either pass the potatoes and pumpkin through a potato ricer or mash the potatoes and pumpkin until smooth.
- Slowly mix in the flour until you form a soft dough.
- Cut off ¼ of the dough and roll into a 1-inch-thick rope. Use the remaining dough to make 3 more ropes.
- Cut each rope into ½-inch segments, and pinch the sides of each piece of dough so it looks like a bow tie. Place the finished gnocchi on a floured pan.
- Freeze the gnocchi for 1 hour.
- Near serving time, bring at least 1 gallon of salted water to a boil. Add half of the gnocchi.
- Cook for 5–6 minutes until the gnocchi float to and remain on the surface for 2 minutes.
- With a slotted spoon, remove gnocchi to a plate, and coat with a little extra-virgin olive oil. Repeat with the remaining gnocchi.

JERUSALEM ARTICHOKE PURÉE

1 leek, cleaned medium dice

4 tbsp olive oil

1 cup peeled Jerusalem artichokes, medium dice

1 cup peeled diced parsnip

Vegetable stock to cover

2 tsp nutritional yeast

Salt and pepper to taste

Fruity extra-virgin olive oil, truffle oil, or nut oil to taste

Fresh grated nutmeg to taste

Fried sage leaves

Chopped parsley

- In a saucepan, sweat the leek in the oil over medium-low until soft.
- Add the artichoke and parsnip. Cover with stock by 1 inch over the vegetables.
- Add the yeast. Simmer, covered, until the vegetables are soft.
- Purée the sauce until smooth in a blender. Adjust salt and pepper.
- Toss the gnocchi in the sauce. Place on a serving plate and drizzle with olive, truffle, or walnut oil.
- Grate nutmeg over the top, crumble fried sage leaves over that, and sprinkle with parsley.

Raw Zucchini and Carrot Lasagna with Almond "Ricotta"

RAVENS' RESTAURANT, MENDOCINO, CALIFORNIA

A true gourmet recipe, ideal for entertaining and showcasing perfectly balanced flavors.

Time: 25 minutes prep; 8 hours to marinate   •   Makes 6 servings

Note: Start this recipe the day before serving or early in the morning: the vegetables need to marinate at least 8 hours. Nutritional yeast, often used in vegan cooking, has a nutty, cheesy flavor. It's available at health food stores.

6 zucchini (about 2 ¾ pounds), trimmed and thinly shaved lengthwise into strips

2 large carrots, trimmed and thinly shaved lengthwise into strips

5 tbsp lemon juice (from about 2 lemons)

5 tbsp olive oil, divided

1 ¾ tsp kosher salt, divided

¾ tsp freshly ground black pepper, divided + more to taste

1 ½ cups raw slivered almonds

3 cloves garlic

2 bunches kale (about 2 pounds), ribs removed, leaves roughly chopped

1 cup lightly packed basil leaves (about 1 bunch)

2 tbsp nutritional yeast (optional)

3 cups baby spinach, cut into thin strips

3 medium tomatoes, cored and roughly chopped

3 medium beets, preferably Chioggia (also called candy-striped) or yellow, peeled and very thinly sliced

Fennel bulb, halved lengthwise, cored, and very thinly sliced

Chopped chervil, or another favorite herb, for garnish

- In a large bowl, toss the zucchini and carrots with the lemon juice, 1 tbsp oil, ¾ tsp salt, and ¼ tsp pepper. Cover and chill. Marinate, gently tossing 2 or 3 times, 8 hours or overnight; drain well, reserving marinade. Meanwhile, put almonds in a large bowl, cover with 2 inches water, and set aside to soak 8 hours or overnight; drain well.
- In a food processor, purée the almonds, garlic, and 2 tbsp oil until smooth; transfer to a large bowl and set aside. In the same processor (no need to clean it), working in batches as needed, pulse the kale and basil, scraping down the sides often, until very finely chopped; transfer to the bowl with the almond mixture. Add the yeast, if using, ½ tsp salt, and ¼ tsp pepper, stirring to combine; set aside.
- Toss the spinach with the reserved zucchini marinade, squeezing with your hands to wilt it; wring dry, and discard marinade. Purée the tomatoes in a blender until smooth; season with ½ tsp salt and ¼ tsp pepper.
- To assemble lasagna, alternate layers of zucchini and carrots with kale-almond mixture and spinach, making 4 layers of each, in a 9" × 13" dish. Arrange beets on top, then scatter fennel over beets.
- Serve immediately, or chill for a few hours first. It can be eaten cold or at room temperature. To serve, pour some of the tomato purée onto each plate, then top with a piece of lasagna. Garnish with chervil and pepper to taste, and drizzle with remaining 2 tbsp oil.

Summertime Succotash with Creamy
Rosemary-Garlic Sauce

One of the most delicious ways to get full, this recipe is ideal for after a long bike ride, when hunger is at its peak.

Time: 40 minutes prep • Makes 4–6 appetizer servings

4 cups zucchini, diced (about 2)

½ tsp sea salt

1 cup shelled fresh or frozen lima beans, blanched for 2 minutes

1 tbsp olive oil or hemp oil

2 tsp lemon juice

1 tsp miso paste

1 garlic clove, mashed

6 sprigs roasemary, for garnish

Black pepper, for garnish

- Using sharp knife, slice the summer squash lengthwise as thinly as possible to form long, flat noodle-like strips. Discard the core area with the seeds as it contains too much moisture. Cut each prepared squash strip into two pieces so that when folded in half, the squash resembles a small ravioli in size.
- Toss the strips with the sea salt. Place in a colander over the sink or a large bowl. Let sit for 30 minutes, rinse, then pat dry.
- To make the filling, place the blanched lima beans, oil, lemon juice, miso paste, and garlic in a food processor and purée until smooth. Set aside until needed.

CREAMY ROSEMARY-GARLIC SAUCE

¾ cup cashews

½ cup water

1 tbsp lemon juice

1 tsp red wine vinegar

¾ tsp minced fresh rosemary

1 large garlic clove

¼ tsp sea salt

- Place the cashews and water in a blender, and process until a thick and smooth cream has formed. Add the remaining ingredients and blend until incorporated.
- To assemble the ravioli, place a small spoonful of the filling mixture on one side a squash strip, then fold over the other side. Pat lightly to seal. Repeat to make the remaining ravioli.
- On each serving plate, pour a small bed of Creamy Rosemary-Garlic Sauce, then place a few ravioli on top. Garnish with a rosemary sprig and black pepper and serve.

Beet Ravioli with Basil Macadamia Ricotta

A fancier dish that is best served as an appetizer. You can also use striped heirloom beets for a stunning presentation, but regular red beets will work as well.

Time: 20 minutes prep • Makes 4–6 appetizer servings

3–4 medium yellow beets, peeled and trimmed
1 cup macadamia nuts
½ tsp sea salt
2 tbsp tahini paste
2 tsp lemon juice
2 tbsp chopped fresh basil
Hemp oil, for garnish
Basil, shredded, for garnish
Freshly cracked black pepper, for garnish

- Shave the beets very thinly into circular rounds by using a mandolin or a sharp knife. Set aside.
- Place the macadamia nuts and sea salt in a food processor, and process until finely ground. Transfer to a small bowl and mix in the tahini, lemon juice, and basil to form a "ricotta."
- For each ravioli, spoon a small portion of ricotta into the center of a beet round, and top with a second beet round, like a sandwich. Once the ravioli have been plated, drizzle with a little hemp oil, basil, and pepper.

Zucchini Pasta with Chunky Tomato Sauce

This zucchini has a classic-style sauce, but the addition of Brazil nuts or walnuts gives it a non-traditional crunch.

Time: 15 minutes active prep • Makes 4 servings

4 medium zucchini
1 tsp + ½ tsp sea salt
20 sundried tomatoes, soaked in warm water until soft (about 30 minutes)
½ cup tomato soak water
2 Roma tomatoes, chopped
1 medium clove garlic
2 heaping tbsp chopped fresh basil
1 heaping tbsp chopped fresh oregano
1 tbsp raisins
1 tbsp hemp oil
½ cup chopped walnuts or chopped Brazil nuts
Pinch red pepper flakes

- Trim the ends of the squash. Using a hand-held vegetable peeler, carefully strip the squash, layer by layer, into noodle-like pieces and gather into a colander (for best results, discard the watery center section that holds the seeds).
- Toss squash strips with 1 tsp of sea salt and place the colander over a large bowl to catch excess moisture. Let rest for 30 minutes.
- After 30 minutes, wash the squash thoroughly with warm water to remove any excess salt, and let drain for 5 more minutes.
- In a food processor, blend together the sundried tomatoes, ½ cup soak water, fresh tomatoes, garlic, basil, oregano, raisins, hemp oil, and ½ tsp of sea salt into a chunky paste.
- Add the nuts and pulse a few times to chop the nuts finely (but do not blend).
- Toss the sauce with the zucchini strips and sauté over medium-low heat for 1–2 minutes to warm through.

Variation: Skip the sauté step and serve at room temperature as a delicious raw dish.

Spaghetti Squash with Three-Step Marinara

Trade in that nutrient-void pasta slopped with a jar of some name-brand red stuff for this fresh and flavorful natural meal. Mesquite and the sweet herb stevia lend a mild sweetness to balance out the acid undertones from the tomatoes, and plentiful fresh herbs bring this dish to life. Served with spaghetti squash, this is a feel-good delicious dinner through and through.

Time: 15 minutes prep; 25 minutes to cook • Makes 2–3 servings as a main dish

2 pounds spaghetti squash (about 1 medium)
1 cups chopped onion
3 medium cloves garlic, minced
2 tbsp coconut oil
3 cups deseeded and chopped tomatoes
   (about 5 medium)
⅛ tsp green stevia or ½ tsp agave nectar

½ tsp mesquite powder (optional)
3 tbsp chopped fresh oregano
2 tbsp parsley + 2 tbsp chopped,
   for garnish
¼ tsp sea salt
½ tsp black pepper

- Cut the squash in half, lengthwise. Place cut side down in a baking pan, and add ½ inch of water to the pan. Bake at 350°F for 40 minutes.
- While squash is cooking, make the sauce. In a large saucepan, sauté the onions and the garlic for about 5 minutes, or until the onions begin to become translucent.
- Stir in all the other ingredients and bring to a boil. Reduce heat to low, and simmer for 20 minutes.
- Place the sauce in a blender and purée until fairly smooth. Return the sauce to the pan, and keep at a low simmer until ready to be served.
- When the squash has finished baking, remove from the oven and allow to cool for a couple minutes. Flip the squash over, and scrape the flesh with a fork to extract the spagetti-like strands from the shell.

To serve
- Place a mound of spaghetti squash on a plate, top with sauce and garnish with parsley. Or combine the squash with the sauce directly in the pan and sauté for 2–3 minutes to reheat and remove any excess moisture.

Note: Do *not* substitute white stevia for the green in this recipe 1:1. White stevia is much sweeter than green. If you choose to use white stevia, add only a tiny pinch to avoid over-sweetening.

Summer Squash Fettuccini with Lemon Pepper Cream

If you make one recipe, make this one: amazingly gourmet tasting, so simple to make. Zucchini can be substituted for the yellow squash. Don't worry about the high quantity of salt—most of it will be washed away.

Time: 15 minutes prep and blend; 1–2 hours to soak cashews; 30 minutes to soak squash; 3 minutes to cook • Makes 6 servings

4–5 medium long yellow summer squash
1 tsp + ¼ tsp sea salt, divided
⅔ cup cashews, soaked in water for 1–2 hours
¾ cup water
1 tsp lemon zest
1 tbsp apple cider vinegar
½ tsp freshly ground black pepper, or more to taste
1 tbsp coconut oil
1 leek, thinly sliced

- Trim the ends of the squash. Using a hand-held vegetable peeler, carefully strip the squash, layer by layer, into noodle-like pieces and gather into a colander (for best results, discard the watery center section that holds the seeds).
- Toss the squash strips with 1 tsp of sea salt and place the colander over a large bowl to catch excess moisture. Let rest for 30 minutes. After 30 minutes, wash the squash thoroughly with warm water to remove any excess salt and let drain.
- Place the soaked, soft cashews in a blender with the water, lemon zest, vinegar, freshly ground pepper, and remaining ¼ tsp sea salt. Blend for several minutes on high until a very smooth cream has formed.
- Heat the coconut oil in a large saucepan over medium heat, then add the leeks. Cook for 2–3 minutes until the leeks have softened. Reduce heat to low and add the blended cream to the pan.
- Stirring constantly, gently warm the mixture for about 1 minute. Add the prepared squash noodles to the pan and toss with the sauce for a just moment until to heat the squash—about 30 seconds to 1 minute.
- Remove from heat and serve immediately, garnishing with additional freshly cracked pepper, if desired.

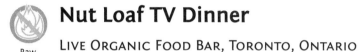

Nut Loaf TV Dinner

LIVE ORGANIC FOOD BAR, TORONTO, ONTARIO

A filling and flavorful loaf, but you'll need a dehydrator for this recipe.

Time: 15 minutes prep; 12–18 hours to dehydrate   •   Makes 4 servings

3–4 cloves garlic
1 red onion
3 ½ cups walnuts, soaked
2 cups pumpkin seeds, soaked
2 cups and 1 tbsp sunflower seeds, soaked
Water to blend
2–3 stalks celery
1 inch ginger, finely chopped
⅛ bunch fresh parsley, chopped
⅛ bunch fresh rosemary, de-stemmed and chopped
¼ tsp cumin seeds
3 tbsp olive oil
¼ tsp Celtic sea salt

- In a food processor, blend the garlic until pasty. Blend the onion until finely chopped.
- Blend the walnuts, pumpkin, and sunflower seeds with a touch of water to blend until smooth, but not too watery; it should be thick. Transfer into a medium-size bowl.
- Finely chop the celery. Add to mixture with remaining ingredients. Adjust salt to taste.
- Form into loaf shape about 4 inches wide and 8 inches long. Cut into ¼-inch slices.
- Lay out onto dehydrator (it is not necessary to use teflex sheets). Dehydrate for 12–18 hours at 115°F until outside is crispy and inside is slightly moist.
- Serve with cauliflower mash potatoes and top with Miso Mushroom Gravy (see p. 210).

Thai Vibe

Raw

LIVE ORGANIC FOOD BAR, TORONTO, ONTARIO

This Thai-inspired noodle salad contains kelp noodles, which are available at local health stores and come ready to eat. Kelp is seaweed high in minerals and vitamins and balances the body's pH levels, among other benefits. Maca will give you fuel for the day. This sauce can be used on pasta or rice as well. Enjoy!

Time: 10 minutes prep • Makes 2–4 servings

MIXED VEGETABLES

½ packages of enoki mushrooms, picked apart
1 bunch of dandelion greens, chiffonade
1 red pepper, julienne
1 red onion, julienne
1 bunch of cilantro, lightly chopped
1 bag kelp noodles
Sunflower sprouts or almonds, for garnish

SAUCE

1 cup of almond butter	1 and ½ Thai chilies or (jalapeños)
2 tbsp chopped ginger	¼ cup of rice vinegar
5 cloves of garlic	½ cup of lime juice
½ red onions	2 tbsp of agave nectar
1 ½ red peppers	1 tbsp of Maca
2 small carrots	Celtic sea salt to taste

- Blend all sauce ingredients together in a blender until smooth.
- In a large bowl, combine all vegetables and the kelp noodles. Add the sauce and toss and serve.
- Garnish with sunflower sprouts or almonds.

Roasted Maple Glazed Brussels Sprouts
with Chestnuts

Delicious and surprisingly filling, this is an ideal side dish to compliment a holiday meal.

Time: 10 minutes prep   •   Makes 6 servings

¼ cup shallots, minced

2 tbsp coconut oil

4 cups Brussels sprouts, halved lengthwise

1 cup chestnuts, roughly chopped, roasted, and peeled
  (fresh, jarred, or vacuum-packed)

1 tsp chopped fresh thyme

¼ tsp each sea salt and black pepper, to taste

1 ½ tbsp maple syrup (grade B)

1 tsp Dijon mustard

1 tbsp apple cider vinegar

- Preheat oven to 425°F.
- In a large roasting pan or ovenproof sauté pan over medium heat, cook the shallots in the oil until soft, about 2 minutes.
- Add the Brussels sprouts, chestnuts, thyme, salt, and pepper and stir well.
- Transfer the pan to the oven and roast for 15 minutes. Remove from the oven and mix in the maple syrup, mustard, and vinegar with the vegetables. Toss well. Return the pan to the oven and continue roasting until the Brussels sprouts are tender, about 10 minutes more.
- Transfer to a serving dish and serve immediately.

Shanghai Rice Bowl

FRESH, TORONTO, ONTARIO

The Shanghai is one of the daily special items on rotation at Fresh. This is a tasty rice bowl that always hits the spot and is easy to prepare.

Time: 10 minutes; 20 minutes for the rice • Makes 2 servings

⅓ cup water
4 baby bok choy, cut in half lengthwise
6 tbsp olive oil
6 tbsp tamari
3 cups shiitake mushrooms, stems removed and halved if large
4 cups cooked brown basmati rice
½ cup Tahini Sauce (see the next page)
2 tsp Mixed Herbs (see p. 233)
2 cups sunflower sprouts
2 tbsp hulled hemp seeds
1 cup cooked or canned chickpeas
2 lemon wedges, for garnish

- Put the water in a wok or skillet over high heat. Add the bok choy halves and cover. Steam 5 minutes until bok choy is almost tender. When water evaporates, add 2 tbsp olive oil, 2 tbsp tamari, and the shiitake mushrooms. Sauté 5 minutes until bok choy and mushrooms are tender. Set aside.
- Divide the cooked rice between 2 large rice bowls, and drizzle both with Tahini Sauce, 4 tbsp olive oil, and 4 tbsp tamari. Sprinkle with Mixed Herbs.
- Place the sautéed bok choy and shiitake mushrooms on the rice, and top with sunflower sprouts, hemp seeds, and chickpeas.
- Garnish with lemon wedges and serve.

TAHINI SAUCE

This is Fresh's most versatile sauce; it tastes great on everything. Tahini, or sesame butter, is made from ground sesame seeds and is high in protein and a good source of essential fatty acids. Tahini is the traditional accompaniment for falafel but can also be used in any kind of stuffed sandwich, as a salad dressing, or as a sauce with rice bowls or noodles.

Time: 5 minutes prep • Makes 4–6 servings

2 cloves garlic, minced
½ cup chopped parsley
½ tsp sea salt
2 tbsp lemon juice
⅔ cup filtered water
½ cup tahini

- In a blender, process the garlic, parsley, salt, and lemon juice until smooth.
- Add the water and tahini, and process until smooth. You may need to add a bit more water if your raw tahini is especially thick. Add water a tablespoon at a time until you get a pourable consistency.
- Store in a sealed container in the fridge for up to 4 days.

Temple Rice Bowl

FRESH, TORONTO, ONTARIO

If we acknowledged and treated our bodies with the same care and consideration as we do a place of worship, we would all be a lot healthier. This is a modest rice bowl that will make you feel good. The hummus, you will discover, goes wonderfully on brown rice.

Time: 10 minutes prep; 20 minutes for the rice • Makes 2 servings

⅓ cup water
4 baby bok choy, cut in half lengthwise
7 tbsp olive oil
4 tbsp tamari
8 wedges tomato
4 cups cooked brown basmati rice
2 tsp Mixed Herbs (see the next page)
1 cup Hummus (see the next page)
2 cups sunflower sprouts
2 tbsp hulled hemp seeds
4 slices red onion, chopped
2 lemon wedges, for garnish

- Put the water in a wok or skillet over high heat. Add the bok choy halves and cover. Steam until the bok choy is almost tender. When water evaporates, add 1 tbsp olive oil, 1 tbsp tamari, and the tomato wedges. Sauté 1 minute until the bok choy is tender, then set it aside.
- Divide the cooked rice between 2 large rice bowls. Mix the remaining 6 tbsp olive oil and 3 tbsp tamari together, then drizzle it over the rice. Sprinkle with Mixed Herbs.
- Place the Hummus in the middle of each rice bowl, and arrange the bok choy around the edge. Top with sunflower sprouts, hemp seeds, and red onion.
- Garnish with lemon wedges and serve.

HUMMUS

This is Fresh's basic hummus recipe. It can be adjusted in countless ways, depending on your preference. You could add parsley or cilantro for an herbal twist, some toasted cumin and cayenne for a bit of spice, or some roasted red peppers, black olives, or sun-dried tomatoes for a Mediterranean taste. If you prefer a milder garlic flavor, roast the garlic before using it.

Time: 5 minutes prep   •   Makes 8 servings

2 cups canned or cooked chickpeas
3 cloves garlic
2 tbsp tahini
4 tbsp lemon juice
½ tsp sea salt
1 tbsp filtered water

- In a food processor, purée all ingredients. Add more water if necessary to get the consistency you like.

MIXED HERBS

This combination of dried herbs adds flavor to many of the recipes at Fresh. The mixture will last forever; just give it a little rub between your fingers before using to release the flavors and aromas. Mixed Herbs are great sprinkled on salads, pastas, noodles, or rice bowls, and keep indefinitely in a sealed jar.

Time: 5 minutes prep   •   Makes 6 tablespoons

1 tbsp dried oregano
1 tbsp dried basil
1 tbsp dried marjoram
1 tbsp dried dill
1 tbsp dried thyme
1 ½ tsp dried rosemary
1 ½ tsp dried sage

- Combine all ingredients in a bowl. Mix well.

Millet Bowl with Greens and Toasted Sunflower Seeds

A macrobiotic-inspired dish with a perfect balance of flavors.

Time: 45 minutes prep • Makes 4–6 servings

1 cup millet, uncooked
3 cups water
1 tbsp miso paste
¼ cup hulled sunflower seeds
1 tbsp coconut oil
1 leek, white and light green parts only, thinly sliced
1 clove garlic, minced
1 tbsp fresh lemon juice
2 cups packed baby spinach
2 cups packed Swiss chard, stems removed and cut into ½ inch strips
Pinch red pepper flakes
Sea salt and black pepper, to taste

- In a dry sauté pan over medium heat, toast the millet for 2–3 minutes, until fragrant. Bring the water to a boil, stir in the miso paste. Reduce heat to a simmer, then add the millet. Cook, uncovered, until water has absorbed, about 30 minutes. Fluff with a fork and keep warm.
- Toast the sunflower seeds over medium heat in a dry skillet for 2–3 minutes, until golden brown and fragrant. Stir constantly to ensure even cooking and to prevent burning. Remove from pan and set aside.
- Heat the coconut oil in a large skillet and add the leek. Cook for 2 minutes to soften, then add the garlic and cook for 30 seconds longer. Add the lemon juice, spinach, Swiss chard, red pepper flakes, and salt and pepper to taste. Reduce heat to medium low, cover the pan, and cook for 5 minutes or until vegetables have wilted and are bright green.
- To serve, place the vegetables on top of the millet and sprinkle with toasted seeds.

Italian Garden Stir Fry

Herb-rich flavors give this stir fry a burst of freshness.

Time: 15 minutes prep • Makes 4–6 servings

1 tbsp coconut oil
½ onion, chopped
2 cups chopped zucchini
1 cup chopped mushrooms
2 cloves garlic, minced
15 ounces cooked garbanzo beans
1 large tomato, puréed (about ½ cup liquid)
1 tsp palm sugar
1 lemon, cut into wedges
2 tbsp chopped fresh mint
1 tbsp chopped fresh oregano
2 tbsp chopped fresh parsley, plus more for garnish
Salt and pepper, to taste
Cooked brown rice or quinoa for serving

- Heat the coconut oil over medium heat in a large cooking pan. Add the onion, zucchini, and mushrooms, and cook for 3–4 minutes until softened.
- Add the garlic and cook for 1 minute longer, then add the beans, tomato purée, and sugar, and squeeze in the juice from half of the lemon wedges.
- Bring to a simmer, then reduce heat to medium low and mix in the fresh herbs. Cook until the liquid has reduced, about 5–10 minutes.
- Add the remaining juice from remaining lemon wedges, remove from heat, and season with salt and pepper, to taste. Serve over a warm bed of rice or quinoa.

Eggplant Rollatini

To save time, make the filling and sauce while the eggplant is cooking (sauce is optional). Other lentils may be used in the place of red lentils—the red lentils are simply more elegant looking. Very filling.

Time: 1 hour prep   •   Makes 4 servings (1 cup of sauce)

2 eggplants
½ tsp sea salt

FILLING

1 tbsp coconut oil
2 cups cooked red lentils (unsalted;
   see p. 181)
1 tbsp miso paste
3 tbsp tahini
2 tbsp fresh minced oregano
2 tbsp fresh minced basil
2 tbsp fresh squeezed lemon juice
2 cloves garlic, minced

SAUCE

1 cup sundried tomatoes, soaked
   in warm water for 20 minutes
1 cup chopped tomatoes
¼ tsp salt
2 garlic clove
2 tbsp chopped fresh basil
1 date
2 tbsp shallot, minced

- Cut off the ends of the eggplant. With a flat end down on the cutting board, slice into ¼-inch strips. Place in a bowl and toss with ½ tsp sea salt to help extract some of the bitterness. Let rest for 10 minutes, then wash thoroughly and pat dry.
- Heat oven to 350°F. Lay the eggplant strips flat on a baking sheet and brush with coconut oil. Alternatively, a coconut oil cooking spray may also be used. Bake for 15 minutes, remove from oven, and let rest until cool enough to handle.
- Meanwhile in a medium bowl, mix together all the filling ingredients. Set aside.
- Blend all sauce ingredients together in a blender until fully combined.

To serve
- Spread 1 cup of the sauce on a baking dish. On a separate work surface lay each eggplant strip flat and spread a heaping tablespoon of filling across each. Roll up into a cylinder and place atop of the bed of sauce.
- Pour the remaining sauce on top and cover with aluminum foil. Bake for 30 minutes, until heated through and the sauce is bubbly.

Quinoa Pilaf with Swiss Chard and Lemon

Macrobiotic-inspired with the additional flavor of garlic.

Time: 5 minutes prep; 20 minutes to cook and sit • Makes 4–6 servings

4 cups water
2 cups quinoa
1 large bunch Swiss chard (about 1 pound)
2 tbsp coconut oil
2 large cloves garlic, minced
2 tbsp minced shallot
1 ½ tbsp lemon zest (grated lemon peel)
½ tsp sea salt, to taste

- Bring the water to a boil and add the quinoa. Cover and cook for about 15 minutes until the water has evaporated. Uncover, fluff with a fork, and let stand for 5 minutes.
- Meanwhile, trim the stems off the chard. Roll leaves together into a large cigar shape and cut into ½-inch slices.
- Heat the oil over medium heat. Add the garlic and shallot, and cook for 1 minute, stirring constantly. Turn the heat to low, add the chard and toss well, then cover and cook for 2 minutes.
- Remove from heat and add the mixture to the quinoa. Add the salt and lemon zest and stir to combine. Serve warm.

Wild Rice with Kabocha Squash and Sage Butter

This is one of my top five recipes, period. It's the perfect fall meal.

To save time, make the rice and butter while the squash is cooking. Yams may also be used in place of the kabocha.

Time: 1 hour prep; 30–45 minutes for the rice • Makes 4 servings

1 pound kabocha squash (about ½ medium squash)
3 tbsp melted coconut oil + 1 tbsp, divided
½ cup wild rice
½ cup brown rice
2 cups water
½ tbsp chopped fresh sage, packed
1 tbsp minced shallots
½ tsp salt

- Preheat the oven to 400°F. Cut the squash in half, then scoop out and discard the seeds.
- Use 1 tbsp coconut oil to lightly brush the cut areas of the squash, and place cut side down on a baking sheet. Bake for 40–45 minutes or until soft when pierced with a fork.
- When cool enough to handle, cut into 1-inch chunks (skin may be left on for extra flavor and nutrition or disposed of). Keep warm.
- To make the rice, combine the rices and water in a saucepan. Bring to a boil, reduce heat to low, and let simmer, covered, until done.
- Meanwhile, in a food processor, blend 3 tbsp coconut oil, sage, shallots, and salt until smooth.

To serve
- In a large pan, heat the sage butter mixture over medium-low heat for 1 minute. Add the rice and toss to combine, and cook for 1 minute longer while stirring constantly. Remove from heat and carefully fold in the squash.

Spicy Black Bean Chili

BLOSSOMING LOTUS, PORTLAND, OREGON

The ideal winter meal.

Time: 15 minutes prep • Makes about 6 2-cup servings

3 tbsp sunflower oil
1 cup diced red onion
¼ green bell pepper
½ cup small diced delicata squash
5 tbsp minced garlic
½ cup whole coriander seeds, toasted
1 tomato, crushed
1 tomato, diced
1 quart water
1 ½ tbsp unrefined cane sugar (optional or can use agave nectar)
2 tsp sea salt
2 ½ tsp apple cider vinegar
½ cup cooked sweet corn kernels
2 ½ tbsp ground cumin powder
1 tsp chipotle powder
3 cups cooked black beans
3 tbsp nutritional yeast

- In very large soup pot, heat the sunflower oil on high; add the onion, bell peppers, squash, and minced garlic. Continue to cook 3–5 more minutes, stirring as needed.
- Toast the coriander and grind in blender. Add both cans of tomatoes to soup pot, along with the water, sugar, salt, vinegar, corn, cumin, chipotle, and coriander. Reduce heat to medium.
- Add cooked beans and nutritional yeast. Turn off heat and mix well. Blend 1.5 quarts of chili in blender and mix back in rest of chili.

Raw

Superfood Chia Chili

LIFE FOOD GOURMET, MIAMI, FLORIDA

A nutrient-packed twist on a traditional dish.

Time: 10 minutes; 6 hours to soak the quinoa • Makes 4 servings

¼ cup chia seeds
1 cup water
4 tbsp tomato sauce (optional but highly recommended)
1 handful fresh cilantro, finely chopped
1 handful fresh parsley, finely chopped
¼–½ cup sprouted red quinoa or sprouted buckwheat
2–4 tbsp each celery, tomato, bell pepper, red onion, chopped
2–4 tbsp cold pressed olive oil
1–3 tbsp tomato powder
1–4 tsp chili powder
1–2 tsp cumin
½–1 tsp turmeric
1–3 tsp apple cider vinegar
½ tsp jalapeño flakes (optional)
½–1 tsp of sun dried sea salt

- Combine the chia seeds and ½ cup of warm water in a bowl and mix thoroughly. Add the remaining ingredients, including the remaining ½ cup of water.

West African Yam and Bean Patties

Just as filling as most burgers, and better tasting too.

Time: 30 minutes prep   •   Makes 8 patties

1 tbsp coconut oil + extra for frying
1 onion, diced
1 pound yams, diced
1 carrot, grated
4–5 cloves garlic, minced
½ tsp ginger powder
2 tsp paprika

¼ tsp cayenne pepper
1 can pinto beans, drained and rinsed
1 cup cooked brown rice
¼ cup quinoa flakes
¼ cup finely chopped almonds
Sea salt and pepper, to taste
Lime wedges, for garnish

- Heat 1 tbsp of coconut oil in a skillet over medium-high heat. Add the diced onion, reduce the heat to medium, and cook until the onions are soft and translucent, about 3–5 minutes. Stir in the yams and add a pinch of sea salt. Cover and cook until the yams are completely tender, about 5 minutes, stirring occasionally. Add the garlic, ginger powder, paprika, and cayenne and cook until fragrant, about 30 seconds. Remove from heat.
- Empty the pinto beans into a large bowl, and use a fork to mash them. Add the cooked vegetable mixture along with the cooked rice, quinoa flakes, and almonds. Stir to combine and then add salt and pepper, if desired. Hand-shape the mixture into 8 patties.
- Heat a small spoonful of coconut oil in a pan over medium-low, then set a couple of patties in the hot pan. Cook the patties for about 6 minutes, then flip them over—you should see a nice crust on the cooked side. If they break apart during the flipping, just reshape them with the spatula—they'll hold together once the second side is cooked. Cook the second side for another 6 minutes. Repeat until all patties are cooked.
- Serve the patties on your bun of choice or atop a bed of greens à la "protein style," with a lime wedge on the side for garnish.

Tip: Chop the yams coarsely, then use a food processor to pulse them into a fine dice.

Fajita Patties

With a bit of a Mexican bite, these "burgers" are a departure from the usual.

Time: 35 minutes active prep • Makes 4–6 servings

1 medium red bell pepper, shredded
1 medium green bell pepper, shredded
2–3 tbsp coconut oil, for frying
1 medium onion, diced (about 1 cup)
2 cloves garlic, minced
2 tsp cumin powder
½ tsp chili powder
¼ tsp cayenne pepper
½ tsp sea salt
1 cup cooked quinoa
¼ cup finely chopped walnuts
¼ cup sprouted flax powder (or finely ground flaxseeds)
2 tsp palm sugar
Lime wedges

- Place the red and green bell peppers in a colander, and squeeze firmly to remove excess liquid (try to get the peppers as dry as possible for best results). Set aside.
- In a medium frying pan, heat 1 tbsp coconut oil over medium-high heat. Add the onion, reduce heat to medium, and sauté for 3–5 minutes or until onions begin to turn translucent. Add the peppers, garlic, cumin, chili powder, cayenne, and sea salt, then cook for 2 minutes longer, stirring frequently. Remove from heat and transfer to a large bowl.
- To the cooked vegetable mixture add the quinoa, walnuts, flax powder, and palm sugar, and mix well. Hand-shape into 4–6 patties.
- Heat a small amount of coconut oil in a large frying pan over low heat. The lower the heat the better, as it will allow the patties to cook longer and get a better crust. Place the patties on the pan carefully, and cook until browned underneath, about 10 minutes. Flip the patties over and repeat on the other side.
- Just before serving, drizzle with fresh lime juice from the lime wedges.

Homestyle Lentil Patties

The classic lentil burger.

Time: 30 minutes active; 50 minutes total • Makes 4–6 servings

2–3 tbsp coconut oil, for frying
1 cup chopped onions (about 1 medium)
1 carrot, shredded
1 celery stalk, minced
1 ½ tbsp balsamic vinegar
1 cup cooked red lentils (see p. 181)
2 tbsp sunflower seeds
¼ cup sprouted flax powder (or finely ground flaxseeds)
Sea salt and black pepper, to taste

- In a medium frying pan, heat 1 tbsp coconut oil over medium-high heat. Add the onions, carrot, and celery, and sauté until the onions are translucent and the vegetables are soft. Mix in the vinegar, remove from heat, and transfer to a large bowl.
- To the vegetable mixture, add the remaining ingredients and mix well, mashing the lentils slightly with a fork. Adjust salt as needed. Place in the refrigerator for 20 minutes to allow the flaxseed to help firm the mixture. Hand-shape into 4–6 patties.
- Heat a small amount of coconut oil in a large frying pan over low heat. The lower the heat the better, as it will allow the patties to cook longer and get a better crust. Place the patties on the pan carefully, and cook until brown underneath, about 10 minutes. Flip the patties over and repeat on the other side. Serve warm.

Indian-Spiced Lentil Hemp Patties

Nutrition-packed and with a unique flavor, these burgers will satisfy a large appetite.

Time: 30 minutes prep • Makes 4–6 patties

2–3 tbsp coconut oil, for frying
1 cup diced yellow onion (about 1 medium)
1 stalk celery, minced
1 cup diced red pepper
6 medium cloves garlic, minced
¼ tsp ginger powder
1 tsp coriander powder
1 tsp cumin powder
½ tsp turmeric
½ cup hemp seeds
3 tbsp sprouted flax powder (or finely ground flaxseeds)
1 ¼ cups cooked red lentils (see p. 181)
½ tsp sea salt, or to taste

- In a medium frying pan, heat 1 tbsp coconut oil over medium-high heat. Add the onion, celery, and red pepper, and sauté until the onion is translucent and the vegetables are soft. Add the garlic and sauté for 1 minute longer. Remove from heat and transfer to a large bowl.
- To the vegetable mixture, add the remaining ingredients and mix well, mashing the lentils with a fork. Adjust salt as needed. Hand-shape into 4–6 patties.
- Heat a small amount of coconut oil in a large frying pan over low heat. The lower the heat the better, as it will allow the patties to cook longer and get a better crust. Place the patties on the pan carefully, and cook until brown underneath, about 10 minutes. Flip the patties over and repeat on the other side. Serve warm.

Chia Bean Patties

Loaded with omega-3-rich chia and mineral-rich wakame sea vegetables, these burgers are a nutritional powerhouse. They can also be cooked, then gently warmed as needed.

Time: 10 minutes prep (once beans are cooked, or use canned); 20 minutes to soak
Makes 8 burgers

2 cups cooked black beans (unsalted)
1 ½ cups cooked brown rice
⅓ cup chia seeds
¼ cup nutritional yeast
1 ½ tsp fresh oregano, minced (or ½ tsp dried)
1 tsp palm sugar
1 stalk celery, minced
1 carrot, minced
½ cup minced yellow onion
3 tbsp brown rice miso
¼ cup quinoa flakes

- With a potato masher or the back of a fork, mash the black beans in a large bowl into a chunky purée. Mix in the remaining ingredients, one at a time. (Alternatively, pulse ingredients together in a food processor, allowing some chunks to remain.) Form into 8–10 patties and refrigerate for 1 hour.
- Heat a spoonful of coconut oil in a large non-stick frying pan over medium-low heat. Add a few of the patties and cook for several minutes on each side until both sides are brown (the finished patties will be crispy on the outside and soft on the inside).

To serve
- Place burgers on sprouted-grain buns with your favorite toppings or "protein-style" in a collard-green leaf.

Variation: Soak 2 tbsp dried wakame flakes for 20 minutes. Drain and mash into the mixture before cooking. Wakame adds an extra-strong punch of trace minerals and a light savory flavor.

Black Bean Sliders

Try serving on a crispy cracker or onion bread with a wedge of avocado.

Time: 10 minutes active; 30 minutes to sit
Makes 2 servings (8–10 small patties)

1 tbsp olive oil
3 large cloves garlic, minced
1 cup diced yellow onion (about ½ medium onion)
1 cup diced green bell pepper (about ½ pepper)
15 ounces cooked black beans (made fresh or canned)
3 tbsp chia seeds
2 tbsp chopped walnuts (optional)
1 cup cooked brown rice
¼ cup quinoa flakes
2 tbsp pumpkin seeds
2 tsp chili powder
1 tsp cumin powder
¼ tsp cayenne powder
2 tbsp nutritional yeast
1 ½ tbsp yacon syrup
Salt, to taste

- Heat the oil over medium heat. Add the garlic, onion, and bell pepper.
- Cook until the vegetables have softened, about 5 minutes. Remove from heat.
- Mix in remaining ingredients. With a fork or simply by hand, mash down the beans to form a chunky mixture.
- Place in the refrigerator, covered, for 30 minutes to allow chia seeds to swell and absorb the excess moisture.
- Form the mixture into 8–10 small patties (sliders). Coat a frying pan with a small amount of oil (olive oil or coconut). Over medium heat, cook the patties for about 5 minutes on each side or until browned.
- Alternatively, place sliders in a pan and cook in the oven with the setting on broil for 5–8 minutes or until just beginning to brown.

Portobello Patties

Full of flavor, these plant-based burgers are extremely versatile.

Time for cooked method: 10 minutes prep; 2–3 minutes to cook • Prep time for raw method: 10 minutes; 10–12 hours to dehydrate • Makes 4 burgers

½ cup ground flax seeds
¼ cup hemp seeds
2 tbsp fresh parsley, chopped
½ tsp fresh thyme, chopped
1 tbsp EFA oil
2 tbsp brown rice miso paste
1 tsp pressed garlic
½ tsp black pepper

2 tbsp nutritional yeast
2 tsp Dijon mustard
¼ cup chopped walnut pieces
2 medium Portobello mushrooms, chopped into large cubes
⅓ cup quinoa flakes (for cooked method only; omit for raw method)

- In a food processor, combine all ingredients except walnuts and mushrooms, and process until well combined. Turn off the processor and add in the walnuts and mushrooms.
- Pulse just 3 or 4 times until the mushrooms are diced, but do not blend. Remove mixture from the processor and transfer to a medium bowl.

Raw method (best)
- Shape the mixture into 4 balls and flatten into patties on a teflex or nonstick sheet. Dehydrate for 10–12 hours at 115°F, then flip and transfer to a mesh sheet and "cook" for 2 more hours.
- These keep for several days wrapped and refrigerated, and can be reheated as needed.

Cooked method
- Mix the quinoa flakes into the mushroom mixture and let stand for 20 minutes.
- Sauté the chopped mushrooms in a dry pan for 2 or 3 minutes to cook out some of the moisture. Follow the rest of the recipe to form burgers.
- To cook, shape the mixture into 4 balls (press firmly to compact) and form into patties. Over very low heat, oil the pan with 1 or 2 tbsp coconut oil.
- Add the patties, and cook approximately 10 minutes on each side. The patties will remain soft on the inside but utterly enjoyable.

To serve
- Try "protein style" on a salad with a mustard vinaigrette, in a collard green with avocado and vegetables, or in a wrap or bun of choice with all the trimmings.

Pizza

The following pizzas are unique in that their crusts are made from legumes and vegetables as opposed to flour; therefore, their crusts are protein and nutrient packed.

Time: 15 minutes prep; about 45 minutes to cook
Makes 1 large pizza (4 servings)

Follow this procedure for all the pizza recipes

- Preheat oven to 300°F. In a food processor, process all crust ingredients until mixture starts to ball up. Lightly oil the baking tray with coconut oil. Spread mixture on tray to about ¼-inch thick (it can be thicker or thinner if you prefer).
- Choose a pizza sauce from the "Spreads, Dips, Sauces, and Dressings" section.
- Bake for 45 minutes. (This will vary slightly depending on the moisture content of the vegetables and the desired crispness of the pizza.)

Buckwheat Sunflower Seed Carrot Pizza

The crust of this pizza is lighter tasting, with a distinct carrot flavor. Choose a pizza sauce from the "Spreads, Dips, Sauces, and Dressings" section.

Time: 15 minutes prep; about 45 minutes to cook
Makes 1 large pizza (4 servings)

CRUST

1 cup ground sunflower seeds
1 cup raw buckwheat
1 cup grated carrot
¼ cup coconut oil
½ tsp parsley
Sea salt, to taste

TOPPING

1 tomato, sliced
½ Spanish onion, diced
1 cup chopped celery
½ cup chopped fresh basil
½ cup grated carrot
½ cup chopped green onions

- Preheat oven to 300°F.
- In a food processor, process all crust ingredients until mixture starts to ball up.
- Lightly oil the baking tray with coconut oil. Spread mixture on tray to about ¼-inch thick (it can be thicker or thinner if you prefer).
- Top with your choice of sauce.
- Spread toppings evenly on the crust.
- Bake for 45 minutes.

Black Bean Chili Pizza

Fiber rich and nutrient dense, this one will end hunger. Choose a pizza sauce from the "Spreads, Dips, Sauces, and Dressings" section.

Time: 15 minutes prep; about 45 minutes to cook
Makes 1 large pizza (4 servings)

CRUST

1 ½ cups cooked brown rice
1 ½ cups black beans
¼ cup coconut oil
1 tbsp chili powder
1 tsp chili flakes
Sea salt to taste

TOPPING

1 tomato, sliced
½ onion, diced
1 cup chopped bell peppers (any color)
½ cup grated beet
½ cup chopped green onions
1 tsp oregano (or 1 tbsp fresh)
1 tsp thyme (or 1 tbsp fresh)

- Preheat oven to 300°F.
- In a food processor, process all crust ingredients until mixture starts to ball up.
- Lightly oil the baking tray with coconut oil. Spread mixture on tray to about ¼-inch thick (it can be thicker or thinner if you prefer).
- Top with your choice of sauce.
- Spread toppings evenly on the crust.
- Bake for 45 minutes.

Quinoa Falafels

Nutrient and flavour packed, these falafels are a divergence from the traditional. You can make the lemon tahini sauce while the falafels are cooking.

Time: 30 minutes prep • Makes about 1 dozen

3 tbsp flax powder
⅓ cup water
2 cups cooked quinoa
3 tbsp nutritional yeast
2 tsp miso paste
1 tsp tahini
1 tsp onion powder
½ tsp garlic powder
¼ cup minced parsley
1 tsp minced fresh oregano
2 tbsp melted coconut oil
Lemon Tahini Dipping Sauce (see p. 202)

- Mix together the flax powder and water in a small bowl and let rest for 10 minutes to form a gel.
- Meanwhile, heat the oven to broil. In a medium bowl, combine quinoa, nutritional yeast, miso paste, tahini, onion powder, and garlic powder, and mix well. Add the flax gel, along with the parsley and oregano, and combine thoroughly.
- To make the falafels, roll a heaping tablespoon of the mix into a ball and flatten into a 2" circle.
- Line a baking tray with aluminum foil, and brush with 1 tbsp coconut oil where the falafels will sit. Place the falafels on the tray, and brush the tops with the remaining tablespoon of melted coconut oil. Put the tray in the oven, and broil for 8 minutes.
- Remove from the oven, flip the patties with a spatula, and return to the oven for another 5–7 minutes, or until patties have formed a dark brown crust.
- Let cool for 1 minute before serving. Enjoy with Lemon Tahini Dipping Sauce on the side or drizzled on top.

Live Falafels

Blossoming Lotus, Portland, Oregon

Enzyme packed, filling, and delicious, but you will need a dehydrator for this recipe.

Time: 15 minutes prep; overnight to soak nuts and dehydrate
Makes about 4 servings

6 tbsp Brazil nuts (soaked overnight)
1 ½ tbsp raw tahini
½ cup dry walnuts
1 scallion, chopped
1 tbsp fresh lemon juice
½ of 1 medium-size jalapeño pepper, seeded and rough chopped
½ cup cilantro
½ cup parsley
1 tbsp dried oregano
1 tsp ground cumin
Salt and pepper, to taste
3 tbsp water, as needed

- Soak the Brazil nuts overnight.
- In blender, purée all ingredients except nuts, and transfer to large bowl.
- In food processor, chop the walnuts into fine mixture and add to the bowl with the puréed ingredients. Drain the Brazil nuts and chop in the food processor. Add to the bowl.
- Thoroughly mix all ingredients. Use a small scoop to make round balls and place on dehydrator sheets.
- Dehydrate for 1.5 hours at 115°F, then turn down to 90°F and dehydrate overnight.

Gorilla Food Green Tacos

GORILLA FOOD, VANCOUVER, BRITISH COLUMBIA

Raw

A filling and satisfying raw taco.

Time: 5 minutes prep (once Walnut Chili Pâté, Salsa, and Guacamole are made)
Makes 4 tacos

4 Romaine lettuce leaves
1 ¼ cup Walnut Chili Pâté (see p. 197)
1 ¼ cup Guacamole (see p. 201)
16 tbsp Salsa (see p. 202)

- Cut just the very bottom off the romaine lettuce bunch so that the leaves fall apart.
- Wash the leaves and pat dry to be used as your taco shells.
- Spread a wide base of Walnut Chili Pâté down the center of each leaf.
- Top the pâté evenly with Guacamole, leaving the pâté visible on the sides.
- Top the Guacamole with Salsa, leaving both the guacamole and pâté visible on the sides.
- Plate and enjoy eating these with your hands.

Whole Foods Recipes   253

Collard Green Buckwheat Wrap

This nutrient-dense wrap is surprisingly filling. For the dressing, choose any in the "Spreads, Dips, Sauces, and Dressings" section.

Time: 10 minutes prep • Makes 1 large serving

1 avocado
2 Roma tomatoes
1 cucumber
1 large carrot
2 strips dulse (about ¼ cup, tightly packed)
1 cup sprouted or cooked buckwheat
1 leaf collard green
3 tbsp salad dressing

- Peel and cube the avocado, slice the tomatoes and cucumber, and grate the carrot. Along with the dulse and buckweat, place on a collard green.
- Drizzle salad dressing over top. Roll up, tucking the ends in so the wrap is secure. Cut into pieces if desired.
- A collard green leaf also serves as a good wrap for guacamole combined with quinoa, buckwheat, or brown rice.

Variation: To serve as a complete meal, add ½ cup black-eyed peas and ½ tsp cayenne pepper to the mixture to spice it up.

Spicy DLT Sandwich

DLT = dulse, lettuce, tomato

Strips of dulse sea vegetables makes this a flavor- and nutrient-packed sandwich. You can use rice bread for a gluten-free option.

Time: 10 minutes prep • Makes 1 serving

2 slices sprouted bread (such as Ezekiel Sesame), lightly toasted if desired
½ avocado, mashed
1–2 tbsp fresh salsa (amount depends on spice level)
¼ cup dulse strips (or 1 ½ tbsp dulse flakes)
Lettuce leaves
Tomato slices

- Toast the bread if desired. Spread the avocado on one side and the salsa on the other.
- Distribute the dulse evenly atop the avocado, stack with lettuce and tomato, and put the sides together.

vegetables

Butternut Squash Soup

KARYN'S ON GREEN, CHICAGO, ILLINOIS

Can be served as a creamy and delicious meal, or in a smaller portion as a complement to a salad. Ideal in the fall.

Time: 5 minutes prep; about 90 minutes to cook • Makes 4 servings

SOUP

2 whole butternut squash (about 5 pounds)
2 cans (about 28 ounces) of coconut milk
Salt, to taste

- Cut tops off the squash and discard. Cut squash in half, lengthwise, and de-seed, saving excess squash for stock. Place halved squash, cut side down, on sheet trays lined with parchment paper. Roast in 350°F oven for about 1 hour or until largest squash is soft throughout.
- Cool to room temperature. Remove the skin from the roasted squash and put the squash in a large sauce pot. Combine coconut milk with squash.
- Simmer squash and coconut milk, stirring occasionally until mixture is heated throughout.
- Remove from heat and use a blender to process mixture on high until smooth. Season with salt to taste, then strain through fine-mesh sieve.
- Pour about 1 cup of soup into each of 4 bowls. Top with some chickpeas and garnish with paprika.

CHICKPEAS

¼ cup canned chickpeas, strained
Oil

½ tsp paprika + some for garnish
Salt to taste

- In fryer at 325°F (or in sauce pot with 325°F oil), fry chickpeas until they begin to brown. Strain excess oil off chickpeas, then toss with paprika and salt in mixing bowl.

Caramelized Brussels Sprouts with Mustard Vinaigrette

KARYN'S ON GREEN, CHICAGO, ILLINOIS

An ideal complement for soup and a salad.

Time: 5 minutes prep; 20 minutes to cook • Makes 4 servings

MUSTARD VINAIGRETTE

1 shallot, minced
2 sprigs of tarragon, chopped
¼ cup champagne vinegar
1cup whole-grain mustard
Lemon juice and salt to taste

- Whisk all vinaigrette ingredients together. Thin with water if desired.

CARMELIZED BRUSSELS SPROUTS

1 pound blanched Brussels sprouts (halved or quartered, depending on size)
Olive oil for sautéing
Salt to taste

- Blanch Brussels sprouts in salted boiling water until al dente. Shock in a bowl of ice water. Drain and pat dry with paper towels. Sear Brussels sprouts in a very hot sauté pan with olive oil until well caramelized. Fold in mustard vinaigrette and season with salt, to taste.

Summary Squash Roast

HORIZONS, PHILADELPHIA, PENNSYLVANIA

Ideal served with a salad, in the summer.

Time: 5 minutes prep; 20 minutes to cook • Makes 6 servings

2 pounds assorted summer squash, seed centers removed
¼ cup of olive oil
1 tsp minced fresh garlic
Salt and pepper
1 cup kalamata olives, pitted and quartered
1 tsp olive oil
1 packed cup fresh basil leaves
1 tbsp vegan sour cream
Pinch salt and pepper

- Preheat oven to 450°F.
- Cut the squash into 1- to 2-inch chunks and toss with ¼ cup of the olive oil, the garlic, salt, and pepper. Roast in the oven for 8 minutes or until just tender.
- Toss the olives in 1 tsp of olive oil and roast in the oven for 12 minutes.
- Purée the basil and sour cream in the food processor. Toss the roasted squash in the basil mixture and garnish with the roasted olives. Add salt and pepper to taste.

Heavenly Baked Delicata Squash

Simple, flavorful squash.

Time: 10 minutes prep; 45 minutes to cook • Makes 4 servings

4 Delicata squash (preferably organic so that you
   can eat the skin and the flesh)
2 tbsp + 1 tbsp virgin coconut oil, divided
1 tbsp dried oregano
½ tsp sea salt or to taste
Freshly cracked pepper, to taste
½ cup water

- Preheat the oven to 400°F.
- Cut off the ends of the squash and slice in half lengthwise. Remove all seeds
  with a spoon and discard. Rub 2 tbsp of coconut oil equally on the insides of
  the squash, and sprinkle evenly with oregano, sea salt, and pepper.
- Place squash cut side down on a large baking tray, and pour ½ cup water in the
  bottom of tray. Loosely cover the tray with aluminum foil or another tray, and
  bake for 45 minutes or until squash is very tender when pierced with a fork.
- To serve, place squash face-up on serving plate, and drizzle with remaining
  tablespoon of coconut oil.

Note: Coconut oil is solid at room temperature but melts quickly. It does not
matter whether the oil is solid or liquid in this recipe, though it may be easier to
distribute when softened or melted.

Turnip Masala

THE GREEN DOOR, OTTAWA, ONTARIO

A new twist on an Indian classic.

Time: 15 minutes prep; 35 minutes to cook • Makes 6–8 servings

8 cups rutabaga, cut into 1-inch cubes
Olive oil and salt for roasting the rutabaga
4 tbsp olive oil
¼ tsp asafetida
½ tsp ground cardamom
½ tsp ground cumin
½ tsp ground turmeric
½ tsp curry powder
1 tsp garam masala
1 tsp ground coriander
3 cloves garlic
1 fresh hot chili pepper (optional)
1 medium onion, diced
2 cups water
1 tsp salt
1 cup diced tomato
½ cup chopped fresh cilantro, for garnish

- Preheat oven to 350°F.
- Toss the cubed rutabaga in a little olive oil and salt. Spread on a baking sheet and bake for 20–30 minutes or until lightly browned and very close to being fully cooked.
- Put a medium-size pot on low heat. Add the oil and all the spices. When they are lightly bubbling, add the garlic and fresh hot pepper. Sauté for 1 minute, then add the onion.
- When the onion is nicely sautéed, add the water. Turn the heat up to high, add the salt and tomato, and bring to a boil.
- Add the roasted rutabaga. Cook for a few minutes, then remove from heat.
- Garnish with fresh cilantro.

Roasted Parsnip with Coconut Fennel Sauce

THE GREEN DOOR, OTTAWA, ONTARIO

An ideal complement to soup.

Time: 10 minutes prep; 35 minutes to cook • Makes 6–8 servings

4 cups parsnip (about 3 regular-size parsnips)
Olive oil and salt for roasting the parsnips
1 tbsp olive oil
2 tbsp freshly ground fennel seed
1 can coconut milk (14 ounces)
Juice of 3 limes
Zest of 1 lime
1 tsp salt, or to taste
Chopped fresh parsley, for garnish

- Preheat oven to 350°F.
- Wash the parsnips. Cut them into chunks averaging 1-inch long, and of roughly equal size so that they roast evenly.
- Drizzle the parsnips with olive oil and lightly sprinkle with salt. Bake for 20 to 30 minutes, or until done.
- Place oil in a large saucepan, add the fennel seed, and roast gently at low heat for 2–3 minutes. Add the coconut milk, lime juice and zest, and salt. Heat slowly, stirring with a wooden spoon.
- When hot, add the roasted parsnip. Adjust salt to taste. Garnish with parsley.

Roasted Cauliflower

Simple, nicely flavored cauliflower.

Time: 5 minutes prep; 45–50 minutes to cook • Makes 2 servings

1 head cauliflower
2–3 tbsp coconut oil, melted
Sea salt
½–1 tsp paprika

- Preheat oven to 375°F.
- Line a baking sheet with parchment paper for easy clean-up.
- Cut the cauliflower into golf ball-size chunks. Toss with the coconut oil, along with the salt and paprika, to taste.
- Spread out evenly on top of prepared sheet and place in the oven for about 40–50 minutes, tossing once halfway through cooking time.

Curried Cauliflower "Rice"

Shredding the cauliflower makes it cook faster and results in a bowl of fluffy vegetable "rice." Simply grate the head of cauliflower with a standard grater using a medium setting.

Time: 10 minutes • Makes 2–4 servings

4–5 cups shredded cauliflower
2 tsp curry powder blend (use your favorite brand or mix)
½ tsp sea salt
1 tbsp coconut oil
1 tbsp apple cider vinegar

- In a bowl, mix together the shredded cauliflower, curry blend, and sea salt.
- In a large skillet, heat the coconut oil over medium heat until melted. Reduce heat to medium and add the cauliflower. Cook, stirring constantly, for about 5 minutes, or until cauliflower is cooked through. Stir in the apple cider vinegar. Remove from heat, and serve.

Mashed Potatoes and Turnips

Like mashed potatoes but more nutritious.

Time: 30 minutes • Makes 6–8 servings

2 quarts water
1 tsp sea salt + additional to taste
1 ½ tbsp palm sugar
3 cups turnips, cut into 1-inch cubes (about 2 medium)
5 cups red potatoes, cut into 1-inch cubes (about 5–6 medium)
1 tbsp coconut oil
2 tbsp nutritional yeast

- Pour the water, sea salt, and palm sugar in a large pot, and bring to a rolling boil.
- Add the turnips and potatoes and cook for 20 minutes, or until tender when pierced with a fork. Drain thoroughly and transfer to a large bowl.
- Add coconut oil and nutritional yeast, and mash into a chunky purée. Serve warm.

Parsnip Oven Fries

Ideal as an autumn meal addition or as a snack, parsnip's "earthy" flavor is brought out by the higher heat of roasting.

Time: 5 minutes prep; 30 minutes to cook • Makes 4 servings

2 pounds of parsnips (about 2–3 large roots)
2 tbsp coconut oil, melted
Salt and pepper to taste

- Preheat oven to 450°F.
- Peel the parsnips and trim the ends. Cut in half lengthwise, then slice into ½-inch sticks. Spread out onto a large baking pan and toss with oil, salt, and pepper.
- Bake for 25–30 minutes or until golden brown, tossing parsnips once or twice during baking to ensure even cooking.

Spicy Cocoa-Hazelnut Zouzous

CRUDESSENCE, MONTREAL, QUEBEC

Zouzous are the Crudessence energy balls.

Time: 10 minutes • Makes about 20 zouzous

3 ½ ounces Brazil nuts
3 ½ ounces hazelnuts
7 ounces (slightly less than ½ pound) sunflower seeds, ground
    to a fine powder with food processor or coffee grinder
¾ cup cocoa powder
⅛ cup agave nectar
2 tbsp maca powder
2 tsp mesquite
1 ½ tbsp carob powder
¼ cup cayenne powder
1 ⅓ cups date paste (make by blending about 2 cups of lightly
    packed pitted dates in a food processor)

- Using the food processor, grind the Brazil nuts and hazelnuts just till they are reduced to a powder, not a butter. Transfer into a large bowl and add the other ingredients, mixing by hand.
- With a small ice cream scoop, form the mixture into balls of approximately ⅛ cup or 2 tbsp per zouzou.

Salt and Vinegar Kale Chips

Crispy, nutrient dense, and flavor packed. These are among the most nutritious and delicious snacks you can make.

Time: 15 minutes prep; cook time varies • Makes 2 medium-size servings or 1 large

½ cup raw sunflower seeds
1 tbsp apple cider vinegar
½ tbsp balsamic vinegar
Water for blending
½ tsp sea salt, to taste
1 bunch curly kale

- Combine the sunflower seeds, both vinegars, and sea salt in a blender. Blend for several minutes until a chunky paste has formed, adding a tablespoon of water into the blender as needed to assist with blending. (The more water that is added, the longer the chips will take in the oven.)
- Strip off the kale leaves into a bowl and discard the stems. Tear up any large pieces roughly, and pour the creamed mixture on top of the kale. Using clean hands, massage the mixture into the kale for one minute to evenly coat the leaves.

Oven method
- Heat the oven to 200°F. Place a piece of parchment paper on top of a baking sheet, then spread out the kale chips evenly over the surface to ensure even cooking time.
- Bake for about 2 hours (time varies according to relative humidity), or until kale has dried out and is crispy. Keep a close eye on the kale at the end of its cooking process to make sure it does not burn.
- Enjoy immediately or keep in an airtight container for up to 2 weeks.

Dehydrator method
- Warm the dehydrator to 115°F. Spread out the kale onto 4 mesh dehydrator sheets, and dehydrate for 10–12 hours, or until crispy (time may vary depending on relative humidity).

Cool Coconut Orange Squares

Easy to make and liked by pretty much everyone.

Time: 45 minutes • Makes about 1 ½ dozen small squares

½ cup cashews
½ cup macadamia nuts
2 large Medjool dates, pits removed
1 tsp orange zest
¾ tsp vanilla extract
½ cup + 2 tbsp shredded dried coconut
¼ palm sugar
Pinch sea salt

- In a food processor, grind the cashews into a coarse flour. Add the macadamia nuts and process until finely chopped. Add in the dates, orange zest, and vanilla extract and mix until dates are combined. Add the remaining ingredients and process until a sticky dough has formed.
- Place a piece of parchment paper or wax paper on a flat surface. Spoon out the dough onto the paper in a mound, and place another piece of paper on top. Use a rolling pin to flatten the dough into a ½-inch-thick layer. Freeze for 30 minutes or longer, till mixture is firm, before cutting into small squares. Best served frozen.

Nori Crisps

Crunchy and fast to make. Since nori burns easily, try baking a small practice batch in the oven to get your timing down.

Time: 10 minutes • Makes about 50 crisps (2–4 servings)

½ tbsp sesame oil
½ tbsp melted coconut oil
½ tsp rice vinegar
1 tbsp palm sugar + extra for sprinkling
¼ tsp sea salt + extra for sprinkling
5 nori sheets

- Preheat oven to 350°F.
- In a small glass or cup, mix together both oils, vinegar, 1 tbsp palm sugar, and ¼ tsp sea salt.
- With a sharp knife or scissors, cut each sheet of nori in half, then cut each half into 5 strips. Lay the strips on a non-stick baking sheet, then lightly brush the surface of the nori with the oil mixture.
- Place in the oven for 3 minutes or until the nori has turned a dark green. Nori burns very easily, so keep a close eye on the time while baking.
- Remove the baking sheet from the oven and lightly sprinkle the strips with additional palm sugar or a bit of sea salt, if desired.

Sour Cream and Onion Kale Chips

Flavor-bursting, nutrient-dense treat.

Time: 35 minutes prep; cook time varies
Makes 2 medium-size servings or 1 large

½ cup cashews, presoaked 35 minutes
⅓ cup water
1 tbsp onion powder
¼ tsp garlic powder
1 ½ tbsp apple cider vinegar
¼ tsp sea salt
2 tbsp minced fresh parsley
1 bunch kale

- Combine the soaked cashews, water, onion powder, garlic powder, vinegar, salt, and parsley in a blender and process until smooth, stopping the machine and scraping down the sides if needed (this may take several minutes). Set aside.
- Wash the kale to remove any grit, then carefully dry the leaves. Strip the leaves into a bowl, roughly tearing any large pieces. Discard the stems. Pour the creamed mixture on top of the kale, using a small spatula or spoon to remove the mixture from the blender. Using clean hands, massage the mixture into the kale for 1 minute to evenly coat the leaves.

Oven method
- Heat the oven to 250°F. Line two baking sheets with parchment paper, then spread the kale chips over the sheets, as evenly and flatly as possible, to ensure even cooking time. Bake between 1 ½ and 2 hours (time varies according to the dryness of the kale), tossing halfway through the baking, until the kale has dried out and is crispy but not burnt. Keep a close eye on the kale at the end of its cooking process, and remove any premature crispy chips from the batch if needed. Enjoy immediately or keep in an airtight container for up to 2 weeks.

Dehydrator method
- Warm the dehydrator to 115°F. Spread the kale onto 4 mesh dehydrator sheets, and dehydrate for 10–12 hours, or until crispy (time will vary depending on relative humidity).

BBQ Red Bell Pepper Kale Chips

Adjust the red pepper flakes to add more or less heat.

Time: 25 minutes prep; cook time varies
Makes 2 medium-size servings or 1 large

1 bunch kale
1 cup red bell pepper, chopped
½ cup water
1 tbsp olive oil
½ cup sunflower seeds

¼ tsp salt
½ teaspoon chipotle powder
1½ tsp onion powder
¼ tsp garlic powder
2 tbsp raisins

- Strip the kale leaves into a bowl, discarding the stems. Tear up any large pieces and set aside.
- Combine all ingredients except for the kale in a food processor or single-serving blender and process until smooth, stopping the machine and scraping down the sides if needed (this may take several minutes).
- Pour the blended mixture on top of the kale, using a small spatula or spoon to remove it from the food processor. Using clean hands, massage the mixture into the kale for 1 minute to evenly coat the leaves.

Dehydrator method (preferred)
- Warm the dehydrator to 115°F. Spread out the kale onto 4 mesh dehydrator sheets, and dehydrate for 10–12 hours, or until crispy (time may vary depending on relative humidity).

Oven method
- Heat the oven to 200°F. Place a piece of parchment paper on top of a baking sheet, and spread the kale chips over the surface, as evenly as possible, to ensure even cooking time.
- Bake for about 75–100 minutes (time varies according to relative humidity) or until kale has dried out and is crispy. For best results, toss the kale several times. Keep a close eye on the kale at the end of its cooking process to make sure it does not burn.
- Enjoy immediately or keep in an airtight container for up to 2 weeks.

Red Raspberry Frozen Fruit Pops

Using stevia is a terrific way to cut down on using sugars. Its sweetness varies from brand to brand, so you'll have to experiment and use it to taste. In this recipe, stevia extends the sweetness of the fruit sugars from date syrup and raspberries without adding a single extra calorie. If you're not a fan of stevia, use another natural sweetener, such as palm sugar or a little extra date syrup.

Time: About 10 minutes; 3 hours to freeze
Makes about 10–12 oz of mixture (servings depend on size of molds)

½ cup unsweetened almond milk
½ tsp vanilla extract
1 cup frozen raspberries
White stevia powder (or liquid), to taste
2 tbsp date syrup

- Get vessels ready for frozen pops—use either a plastic mold or kit, or small cups with sticks.
- In a medium bowl, stir together the almond milk and vanilla. Add the frozen raspberries, and use a fork to "mash" them into the liquid—the milk will begin to freeze into a slush around the raspberries, which is the objective.
- Mix until chunky, but not blended. Add a tiny, tiny dash of stevia and mix well. Taste the mixture and add more stevia if needed, mixing after each addition. The overall taste should be quite sweet, as freezing will bring the sweetness down a notch.
- Drizzle the date syrup into the mixture. Stir once or twice *only*—just enough to incorporate the syrup into the raspberry mix but allowing large date syrup swirls to remain.
- Carefully spoon the mixture into the molds. Freeze for 3 hours or until mixture is completely frozen through. Thaw for a minute or two just before serving.

energy bars and gels

In sharp contrast to conventional energy bars, these bars are true high-net-gain food.

They provide fast and sustained energy, and are easy and quite quick to prepare—no cooking involved. I like to make a big batch once a month, wrapping the bars individually in plastic wrap and freezing them, so that I always have a variety on hand. Because these bars maintain a supple and chewy consistency even when frozen (unlike commercial bars, which freeze rock-solid), you don't need to wait for them to thaw to enjoy them.

Follow this procedure for all the energy bar recipes, unless otherwise stated.

- In a food processor, process all ingredients until desired texture is reached. If you prefer a uniformly smooth bar, process longer. If you would rather a bar with more crunch and texture, blend for less time.
- Generally, if I'm making the bars specifically to be eaten during physical activity, such as long training rides, I'll blend the mixture until it is smooth, as this will reduce the amount of chewing required. However, for variety, I'll also be sure to make a few batches at the same time that are crunchier, to eat as a regular snack.
- Remove mixture from processor and put on a clean surface. There are two ways to shape the bars: you can roll the mixture into balls or shape it into bars.
- To shape into balls, use a tablespoon or your hands to scoop the mixture (however much you like to make one ball), then roll it between the palms of your hands.
- To shape as bars, flatten the mixture on the clean surface with your hands. Place plastic wrap over top, then, with a rolling pin, roll mixture to desired bar thickness. Cut mixture into bars.
- Alternatively, form mixture into a brick, then cut as though slicing bread. As the bars dry, they become easier to handle.

Spiced Açaí Energy Bars

Time: 45 minutes total; 15 minutes active • Makes 8–10 bars

¾ cup raw almonds
¾ cup pitted Medjool dates
  (about 6 large)
3 tbsp açaí powder
2 tbsp raisins
¼ cup dried apricots

1 tbsp chia seeds
½ tsp ginger powder
½ tsp cinnamon powder
¼ tsp vanilla extract
Tiny pinch of salt (optional)

- Mix all the ingredients together in a food processor just until a dough has formed (allowing some almonds to remain coarsely chopped).
- Place a sheet of plastic wrap on a cutting board and spill the dough out on top. Use your hands to press and form it into a 1-inch-thick rectangle.
- Cover the rectangle of dough with plastic wrap and place it in the freezer for 30 minutes, then cut into 8–10 bars. These are best eaten cold, since they're stickier when they're warm.

Green Energy Bars

Chlorophyll-packed, these green bars taste much better than they look.

Time: 15 minutes • Makes 8 bars

1 cup raw cashews
1 cup pitted Medjool dates (about 8 large)
2 tsp wheatgrass powder
¼ cup hemp seeds

- Mix the cashews, dates, and wheatgrass powder together in a food processor just until a coarse dough has formed (allowing some cashews to remain coarsely chopped). Add the hemp seeds and pulse several times until combined.
- Place a sheet of plastic wrap on a cutting board and spill the dough out on top. Use your hands to shape the dough into rectangle about 1-inch thick, then cut into 8 pieces. Wrap and keep in the freezer for long-term storage.

Chocolate Sacha Inchi Blueberry Energy Bars

High in antioxidants and flavonoids, these bars help reduce free radical damage in the body and improve cellular recovery after workout.

Time: 10 minutes • Makes about a dozen 1 ¾ oz bars

1 cup fresh or soaked dried dates
¼ cup sacha inchi seeds
¼ cup blueberries
¼ cup roasted carob powder
¼ cup ground flaxseed
¼ cup hemp protein
¼ cup unhulled sesame seeds
1 tsp fresh lemon juice
½ tsp lemon zest
Sea salt, to taste
½ cup sprouted or cooked buckwheat (optional)
½ cup frozen blueberries
¼ cup chopped sacha inchi seed

- In a food processor, process all ingredients except the buckwheat, blueberries, and chopped sacha inchi seeds. Knead the buckwheat, blueberries, and sacha inchi seed into the mixture by hand.

Walnut Cranberry Energy Bars

High in antioxidants and flavonoids, these bars help reduce free radical damage in the body and improve cellular regeneration.

Time: 10 minutes • Makes about a dozen 1 ¾ oz bars

1 cup fresh or soaked dried dates
¼ cup walnuts
¼ cup fresh or frozen cranberries
¼ cup ground flaxseed
¼ cup hemp protein
1 tbsp coconut palm sugar
¼ cup unhulled hemp seeds
Sea salt to taste
½ cup sprouted or cooked buckwheat (optional)
¼ cup copped walnuts
½ cup frozen cranberries

- In a food processor, process all ingredients except the buckwheat, walnuts, and cranberries. Once the ingredients are well blended, knead in the buckwheat, walnuts, and cranberries into the mixture by hand.

These gels contain coconut oil, which provides direct energy to the liver and dramatically improves endurance when combined with a carbohydrate source. And they contain chia. Chia provides sustained nutrients in an easily digestible whole food form. When the energy from the glucose contained in the dates begins to wear off, the slower-release energy from the maple syrup is activated, followed by the ultra-slow sustained energy release of chia.

The gels take only minutes to make, and can be carried in a standard two-ounce gel flask, available in most running stores.

Carob Energy Gel

2 large Medjool dates

1 tbsp agave nectar

1 tbsp ground chia

1 tbsp coconut oil

1 tsp lemon zest

1 tbsp fresh lemon juice

1 tsp cocoa nibs (or substitute carob powder)

Sea salt, to taste

- Blend all the ingredients together into a gel-like consistency. For an extra kick, add 1 tsp of ground yerba maté.

Lemon Lime Energy Gel

2 large Medjool dates

1 tbsp agave nectar

1 tbsp ground chia

1 tbsp coconut oil

½ tbsp lemon zest

½ tbsp lime zest

½ tsp dulse

Sea salt to taste

- Blend all the ingredients together into a gel-like consistency. For an extra kick, add ½ tsp of ground yerba maté and ½ tsp of green tea.

Raw

Raw Berry Parfait

KARYN'S FRESH CORNER, CHICAGO, ILLINOIS

Simple, raw, and delicious.

Time: 5 minutes active; 6 hours presoak   •   Makes 6–8 servings

2 cups cashews
6 cups purified water
¼ cup agave nectar or sweetener of choice
1 cup ground flaxseed or granola
1 ½ cups thinly sliced strawberries

- Soak cashews for 6 hours in 4 cups purified water. Drain and rinse.
- Blend cashews, 2 cups water, and agave nectar to a creamy consistency.
- In a large bowl or among individual parfait glasses, spoon in a dollop of the cashew cream, cover with a thin layer of granola or flax, then arrange a thin layer of strawberry slices.
- Repeat with one or two more rounds of layers. Best served chilled.

Raw

Banana Nut Bread

BEETS LIVING FOODS CAFÉ, AUSTIN, TEXAS

Making this "bread" requires some planning and a dehydrator, but it's worth the extra effort.

Time: 10 minutes active; 12–16 hours to dehydrate • Makes 12 servings

6 fresh bananas (approximately 20 ounces by weight)
2 cups cored and chopped apple
1 ½–2 cups zucchini, peeled and chopped
¼ cup dried raisins or cranberries
1 cup frozen blueberries or cranberries
2 tsp lemon juice
½ tsp vanilla
1 cup ground chia seeds
½ cup soaked, dehydrated walnuts, chopped

- Place the bananas, apples, zucchini, raisins, blueberries, lemon juice, and vanilla in a food processor outfitted with the S-blade. Process until smooth and pour into a large bowl.
- Add the ground chia seeds. Combine thoroughly with a whisk, making sure to break up any clumps.
- Use a scoop or a ¼-cup measure to "plop" mixture onto a paraflex sheet on dehydrator tray lined with the mesh sheet. Spread lightly into desired shape and sprinkle with chopped walnuts.
- Dehydrate for 6–8 hours.
- Invert onto a different tray. Peel back the paraflex and continue to dry for an additional 6–8 hours.

Raw

Key Lime Pie

CRUDESSENCE, MONTREAL, QUEBEC

A delicious, creamy, raw version of the classic Key Lime Pie.

Time: 20 minutes • Makes 1 pie (serves about 8)

CRUST

1 cup macadamia nuts

1 ½ cups coconut, shredded

⅛ cup date paste

⅛ tbsp sea salt

¼ tbsp vanilla extract

- Using a food processor, process macadamia nuts to a butter. Add the other ingredients and process until the mixture is uniform. Spread over the bottom of a pie pan.

FILLING

6 cups avocado flesh

1 ½ cup lemon juice

1 cup coconut butter

1 cup agave nectar

½ tsp vanilla extract

- Place all ingredients in a blender and blend until well combined. Empty the mixture on top of the crust and spread evenly.

ICING

¼ cup lemon juice

2 cups macadamia nuts

3 tbsp agave nectar

1 tsp vanilla extract

Pinch of sea salt

¾ cup water

3 tbsp coconut oil, melted

- Place all ingredients—*except* coconut oil—into the blender and mix until a smooth uniform liquid without lumps is obtained. Add the melted coconut oil while blender is on; blend till oil is mixed throughout. Carefully spread the icing on top of the filling. Beginning at the center of the pie, create two spiral lines of icing. With a fork, draw the shape of a spider's web. Refrigerate before serving.

Banana Crème Pie

MATTHEW KENNEY

Raw

Delicious raw and liked by all, this pie can be safely served to traditional dessert eaters.

Time: 30 minutes active; 30 minutes to sit • Makes 1 pie

CRUST

1 ½ cups macadamia nuts

½ cup coconut flakes

½ tsp salt

3 tbsp agave syrup

1 tbsp coconut oil

1 tsp vanilla extract (or 1 bean)

- In a food processor, process the macadamia nuts, coconut flakes, and salt until they are crumbly flour. Add the agave, oil, and vanilla, and lightly pulse until all ingredients are well combined but mixture only sticks together when pressed between your fingers.

BANANA CRÈME FILLING

3 cups soaked cashews

2 cups mashed banana

1 cup agave syrup (or ½ cup, with
  ½ cup honey)

2 tsp vanilla extract

1 tbsp lemon juice

¼ tsp salt

½ cup coconut oil

- Blend the first six ingredients until smooth. Add the coconut oil and blend until combined.

COCONUT CRÈME

1 ½ cups soaked cashews

1 ½ cups coconut milk

½ cup agave

1 tbsp vanilla

1 tsp lemon juice

1 cup coconut oil, liquefied

Pinch of salt

1 sliced banana for layering

- Blend the first five ingredients until smooth. Then add coconut oil and salt and continue to blend until completely combined. Chill in the refrigerator for a few minutes before using in order to let it set.

To serve
- Press crust into a 9-inch tart pan with a removable bottom. Pour in banana crème filling. Top with one thinly sliced banana. Top with coconut crème. Let set in the refrigerator for at least 30 minutes before serving.

Cherry Tartlets with Vanilla Crème

CHAD SARNO

Serve this dessert when you want to be fancy and impress.

Time: 15 minutes active; 1 hour to sit • Makes 12–15 tartlets

CRUST

1 cup raw macadamia nuts

1 cup unsweetened, dried,
   fine shredded coconut

¾ cup agave nectar

3 tbsp lemon zest

⅛ tsp sea salt

- In a food processor, process all ingredients until finely ground. The mixture should form into a ball when pressed. Using small 2- or 3-inch tartlet shells, line each with plastic wrap, press 2 tbsp crust mixture into each tartlet shell, then remove the tart from the shell and chill.

VANILLA CRÈME

1 cup cashews (presoaked in water
   4 or more hours to soften)

¼ cup agave nectar

3 tbsp coconut butter

½ cup orange juice

1 whole vanilla bean seeds scraped

1 tbsp lemon zest

1 tbsp lime zest

- In a high-speed blender, blend cashews, agave, coconut butter, juice, vanilla bean, and lemon and lime zest. Chill blended mixture until ready to serve, at least 1 hour.

GARNISH

1 cup pitted whole cherries

Mint sprigs or edible flowers (optional)

LAVENDER SYRUP (OPTIONAL)

¼ cup dried lavender flowers

1 cup agave nectar

1 cup hot water

- Steep the lavender flowers in hot water for 20 minutes, then strain the water and whisk in the agave.

To serve

- Set one tartlet shell in the center of each plate and top with 2 tbsp vanilla crème. Add a little lavender syrup, if you want to be really fancy. Garnish with cherries and mint or edible flowers.

Chocolate-Covered Sacha Inchi Bananas

A nutrient-rich twist on a simple, delicious classic.

Time: 10 minutes active; 5–6 hours to freeze • Makes 8 servings

¼ cup sacha inchi, chopped fine
4 bananas, peeled and halved, frozen for a minimum of 1 hour
1 batch Simple Chocolate Sauce (see below)

- Place the sacha inchi on a plate. Dip the cold banana halves into the sauce, covering as much surface area as possible, then roll in sacha inchi pieces.
- Place the banana piece on a plate and repeat with remaining bananas. Cover the coated bananas loosely and place the plate in the freezer until bananas are frozen through, about 5 hours.

Simple Chocolate Sauce

Use this sauce as a perfect ice cream topping, a dip for cold fruits, or drizzled on top of other desserts.

Time: 5 minutes • Makes ⅔ cup

⅓ cup coconut oil
½ cup cocoa powder
¼ cup agave nectar or maple syrup

- In a small saucepan, melt the coconut oil over low heat until liquid. Add the cocoa powder and agave nectar and whisk to form a smooth sauce.

No-Bake Double Chocolate Chip Maca Cookies

Soft and sweet. The secret is in the toasting of the coconut, which gives these the taste of "baked" cookies. For the chocolate, use the darkest chocolate you can find.

Time: 15 minutes • Makes about 1 ½ dozen

¼ cup shredded coconut
⅓ cup coconut flour
2 tbsp cocoa powder
2 tsp maca powder (gelatinized)
2 tbsp palm sugar
Pinch sea salt
2 tbsp almond butter
½ tsp vanilla extract
¾ cup Medjool dates, pits removed (about 6 large)
1 ¾ ounces dark chocolate, chopped into small chunks

- Heat a small frying pan over low heat and add the coconut. Toast the coconut until it has turned an amber color (about 1 minute), stirring constantly as coconut will burn easily. Remove from heat.
- Place the toasted coconut, coconut flour, cocoa powder, maca, palm sugar, and sea salt into a food processor and start the machine. Add the almond butter and vanilla extract, then, one at a time, add the pitted dates and process until a crumbly dough has formed.
- Stop the machine and check the consistency: the dough should stick together easily between two fingers when pinched. If too wet, add additional coconut flour. If too dry, add water about ¼ tsp at a time until correct consistency is reached.
- Transfer to a bowl and mix in the dark chocolate chunks. Using clean hands, grab a small amount—about a tablespoon—and squeeze and roll to form a tight ball. Flatten the ball using your palm or the back of a glass to form a small cookie.

Mint Chip Ice Cream

With a fresh coconut and strong mint flavor, this ice cream is a favorite.

Time: 10 minutes active; about 6 hours to freeze • Makes about 1 pint (serves 4)

½ cup young coconut meat (about 1 coconut)
1 ¼ cup raw cashews
1 cup water
¾ cup vanilla unsweetened almond milk
⅓ cup fresh mint leaves
⅓ cup + 1 tbsp agave nectar
12–15 drops mint extract
⅓ cup chopped dark chocolate

- Blend the coconut meat, raw cashews, water, almond milk, fresh mint, and agave together into a smooth cream.
- Carefully add the mint extract—a little goes a long way, so take care not to spill. Blend again, taste, and add more extract if desired.
- Transfer to a bowl or Tupperware container and freeze, covered, for 1 hour until chilled. Add in the chopped dark chocolate and mix thoroughly. Return to the freezer and enjoy when frozen through—about 4-6 hours. Let defrost for a couple of minutes to soften slightly before serving.

Vanilla Protein Ice Cream with Caramel Swirl

Time: 10 minutes prep; about 6 hours to freeze • Makes 4–6 servings

ICE CREAM

1 cup cashews

1 cup water

1 banana

1 scoop Vanilla Vega Sport Protein Powder

2 tbsp agave nectar

1 tsp vanilla extract

- Blend the cashews, water, banana, protein powder, agave nectar, and vanilla in a blender until smooth. Transfer to a bowl or Tupperware container, cover, and place in the freezer.

CARAMEL SWIRL

2 tbsp yacon syrup

2 tsp almond butter

Pinch of sea salt

- In a small glass, mix the yacon, almond butter, and a pinch of sea salt together to form a sauce. After the ice cream has frozen for about 1 hour and begun to thicken, fold the sauce into the ice cream—mixing just enough to form caramel swirls (do not fully incorporate). Place the ice cream back in the freezer until frozen—about 5 hours.

Chocolate Chip–Maple Maca Ice Cream

If you have an ice cream maker, feel free to put it to use for a fluffier texture.

Time: 10 minutes active; 6–8 hours to freeze • Makes about 1 pint

1 cup cashews
1 cup water
½ banana
¼ cup maple syrup
2 tbsp gelatinized maca powder
Pinch sea salt
1 tsp vanilla extract
⅓ cup chopped dark chocolate

- Blend all ingredients—except the chopped dark chocolate—in a blender until completely smooth. Transfer to a bowl or Tupperware container and freeze for 30 minutes.
- Mix in dark chocolate chunks into the cold ice cream, then continue freezing, covered, until frozen through—about 6–8 hours.
- Let defrost for 5 minutes to soften before serving.

Cantaloupe Ginger Ice

The ginger flavor is very delicate. Only use fresh. Ginger lovers can add more.

Time: 15 minutes active; about 4 hours to freeze • Makes 4 servings

4 cups cantaloupe flesh (about one medium)
1 ¼ tsp fresh grated ginger
2 tbsp agave nectar (or use white stevia, to taste)

- Combine all ingredients in a food processor, and purée until mostly smooth. Transfer mixture to a shallow bowl or pan, cover, and place in the freezer. About once an hour, use a fork to break up any frozen chunks into a fluffy snow. Repeat until entirely frozen, about 4 hours.

Watermelon Lemon Granita

Granita is an Italian ice. Very refreshing.

Time: 15 minutes active; about 4 hours to freeze • Makes 4 servings

4 cups watermelon flesh, seeds removed
½ tsp lemon zest
2 tbsp lemon juice
1 tbsp agave nectar (or use white stevia, to taste)

- Combine all ingredients in a food processor, and purée until mostly smooth.
- Transfer mixture to a shallow bowl or pan, cover, and place in the freezer. About once an hour, use a fork to break up any frozen chunks into a fluffy snow.
- Repeat until entirely frozen, about 4 hours.

Indigo Granita

The antioxidant powerhouses of blueberries and açaí combine forces to produce a colorful, healthy, and refreshing frozen berry dessert. Serve in a wine glass with a sprig of mint for the full esthetic effect.

Time: 15 minutes active; about 4 hours to freeze • Makes 2–4 servings

1 ½ cups frozen blueberries, partially thawed
¼ cup lemon juice
1 tbsp maple syrup
1 tbsp agave nectar
2 tbsp açaí powder
Touch of stevia, if desired
2 tbsp water + more if needed to blend

- Combine all ingredients in a food processor, and purée until mostly smooth.
- Transfer mixture to a shallow bowl or pan, cover, and place in the freezer. About once an hour, use a fork to break up frozen chunks and fluff into a snow. Repeat until entirely frozen, about 4 hours.

Bodacious Berry Cookie Crumble

Great crumbled on top of ice creams or use as a flavorful pie crust.

Time: 5 minutes • Makes 8- or 9-inch pie crust, depending on thickness

1 cup cashews
8 large Medjool dates, pitted
2 tbsp Vega Shake & Go Bodacious Berry Instant Smoothie Mix
1 tbsp coconut oil

- Grind the cashews into a flour in a food processor. With the machine still running, add the pitted dates, one at a time, until fully incorporated. Add the Smoothie Mix and the oil and process until a dough has formed.

Summery Simple Peach Tart

Best made in the summer with in-season peaches.

Time: 5-10 minutes • Makes 6 tarts

1 cup almonds
¼ cup ground flaxseeds
4 dates
2 tbsp palm sugar
2 tsp vanilla extract
Pinch sea salt
2–3 peaches, chopped
Cinnamon, for garnish
Vanilla or maca ice cream, for serving

- To make the crust, grind the almonds into a flour in a food processor. With the machine still running, add the flax seeds, dates, sugar, vanilla, and sea salt and process until fully incorporated. Press the dough into a tart pan to form a crust and top with peaches and cinnamon.

Variation: Place peaches in individual serving bowls and simply crumble the almond mixture on top. Serve with any ice "cream" recipe from this book.

Yacon Dessert Ravioli

The mild taste and satisfying crunch of reconstituted yacon is complemented by a delectable sweet citrus-spice filling. Serve with a good non-dairy vanilla ice cream, or make the raw version below and keep this recipe 100 percent raw. An impressive gourmet dessert with gorgeous flavor notes that are not to be forgotten!

Time: 10 minutes active; about 6 hours to freeze • Makes 12 ravioli (serves 2–4)

2 cups orange juice, or enough to immerse yacon slices
24 large yacon slices (try to pick larger, rounder slices)
½ cup walnuts
¼ cup raisins
1 ½ tbsp yacon powder
¼ tsp nutmeg
¼ tsp cinnamon
½ tsp orange zest (grated orange rind) + some for garnish
One recipe Vanilla Protein Ice Cream with Caramel Swirl (see p. 284)
Yacon syrup, for garnish

- In a large bowl, pour orange juice over yacon slices until submerged. Allow to reconstitute for 1 hour.
- In a food processor, combine walnuts, raisins, yacon powder, nutmeg, cinnamon, and orange zest. Process until a sticky filling has formed. Remove the mixture from the processor and knead to combine ingredients completely, if necessary.
- Remove yacon slices from orange juice and blot on a paper towel to remove any extra juice. To make the ravioli, place a small teaspoon of the filling in the center of a yacon slice. Top with another yacon slice, and pat the edges slightly to form a ravioli. Repeat until all yacon slices are used.

To serve
- Place 3 or 4 ravioli on a dessert plate, and top with a scoop of Vanilla Protein Ice Cream. Drizzle with yacon syrup and dust with orange zest, if desired.

White Chocolate Raspberry Cheesecake
with Chocolate-Almond Crust

Cacao butter is the secret ingredient to making this phenomenally smooth and sophisticated non-dairy cheesecake. Not only does the cocoa butter perfume the mixture with white chocolate luxury, but it also helps solidify the cheesecake. The cocoa paste has the same effect in the dark chocolate almond crust, which retains a satisfying chocolate crunch because of the hint of cocoa nibs. Mesquite powder enhances the chocolate flavor even further, serving as a natural flavor match for cocoa.

Time: 20 minutes active; 30 minutes to freeze   •   Makes 1 9-inch cheesecake or 6 5-inch mini cheesecakes

CRUST

1 cup raw almonds

1 cup Medjool dates, pits removed (about 8)

2 tsp mesquite powder

3 tbsp melted cocoa paste (approximately ¼ cup unmelted shavings; melt using a double boiler method)

½ tsp almond extract

Pinch sea salt

1 tbsp cocoa nibs

- Use a food processor to blend the almonds, dates, mesquite, cocoa paste, almond extract, and sea salt together into a crumbly dough. Add the cocoa nibs and pulse several times until just combined but not blended through, to retain a bit of crunchy texture.

CHEESECAKE

2 pints fresh raspberries

2 cups raw cashews

3 ½ ounces melted cocoa butter (about 1 cup dry shavings; melt using a double boiler method)

½ cup agave nectar or maple syrup

2 tbsp lucuma powder

4 tbsp vanilla extract

2 tbsp fresh lemon juice

Simple Chocolate Sauce (see p. 281; optional)

Fresh raspberries, for garnish

- Use a blender to purée the raspberries. (If you wish, you may strain the berries to remove all the seeds but retain the liquid, then place the juice back in the blender. If you don't mind a few seeds in the cheesecake, you can skip this step.) To the raspberries, add the remaining ingredients and blend until very smooth (this may take a few minutes).

To serve

- Use a 9-inch springform pan and press the crust evenly across the bottom to form a dense, flat layer. Pour the cheesecake mixture on top.
- Place in the freezer for at least 30 minutes to set; freeze until ready to serve. To serve, drizzle with Simple Chocolate Sauce if you wish, then decorate with fresh raspberries.

Variation: Make mini cheesecakes instead. When the cake components are ready, line six 5-inch ramekins tightly with plastic wrap, allowing extra wrap to flow over on all sides of the ramekin to ease later removal (alternatively, simply use mini-springform molds). Make the mini cakes just as you would the larger one. When ready to serve, simply lift the cheesecakes out of the ramekins by pulling up on the plastic wrap.

Apple-Pear Energy Tartlets

Of course, simply doubling the recipe and making one large tart works too.

Time: 10 minutes • Makes 6 3-inch tartlets

1 medium sweet crunchy apple (Fuji or Gala work well)
1 medium soft pear (Bartlett or Bosc)
½ tsp pumpkin pie spice, or cinnamon
1 tbsp yacon syrup (optional)
3 Vega Whole Food Vibrancy Bars, Original Flavor

- Chop the apple and the pear into a fine mince. Toss with pumpkin pie spice and yacon syrup until well combined. Set aside.
- Using a standard-size muffin tin or tartlet molds, tuck a layer of plastic wrap into one of the cups to use as a mold.
- Break the energy bars into halves. Take one of the bar pieces and press it firmly into the lined cup, coaxing the bar "dough" evenly along the bottom and up the sides about ½ inch with your fingers to form the tartlet base.
- Use the plastic wrap to remove the packed base from the muffin tin, then peel away the plastic. Use the plastic again to form the remainder of the tartlets.
- Liberally spoon in the apple-pear filling evenly into each of the tartlet crusts and serve.

GUIDE TO NUTRIENTS

MICRONUTRIENTS

Phytonutrients

Also referred to as a phytochemical, a phytonutrient is a plant compound that, by boosting the immune system, offers health benefits independent of its nutritional value. As you can see, for "Best sources" I specify "organic" foods. That's because phytonutrients are often the plant's natural pest deterrent, whereas if chemical pesticides are used, the plant won't produce phytonutrients. It's suspected that a vast quantity of phytonutrients—with benefits we aren't even aware of—have yet to be discovered. But it's believed that they will most probably be present in the same foods that contain known phytonutrients.

Best sources: organic vegetables, organic seeds, organic fruit, organic nuts, green tea, yerba maté.

Antioxidants

Antioxidants are naturally occurring compounds, including vitamins C and E and the mineral selenium. Antioxidants are most prized for their ability to protect cells. Helping rid the body of free radicals, antioxidants are credited with helping to maintain cellular health and to promote cellular regeneration. If not for antioxidants, cellular damage caused by stress would advance quickly and likely lead to disease.

Best sources: organic colorful fruits and vegetables, organic berries, organic sweet peppers.

VITAMINS

Vitamin A

Vitamin A helps the body resist infection, which it is more prone to after physical exertion, and allows the body to use its reserves for repairing and regenerating muscle tissue (instead of fighting infection)—leading to quicker recovery. Vitamin A helps support growth and repair of muscle and maintains red and white blood cells—crucial for performance.

Best sources: orange and dark green vegetables, including carrots, pumpkin, sweet potatoes, winter squash, broccoli, kale, parsley, and spinach; apricots, mango, papaya, cantaloupe.

Vitamin B1

Vitamin B1 helps the body convert carbohydrate into energy. Maintaining high energy levels depends in part on maintaining adequate vitamin B1 in the diet. People who eat healthy food rarely have a problem getting enough vitamin B1; it's plentiful in many foods. Also, because active people expend more energy than the average person, they need more vitamin B1. Again, this is usually not a problem, since with increased activity comes increased appetite.
Best sources: legumes, pseudograins, nuts, brown rice, nutritional yeast, and blackstrap molasses.

Vitamin B2

Vitamin B2 helps break down amino acids (protein) for the body to use. Utilization of amino acids is a key factor in quick muscle recovery and regeneration after exertion. Like vitamin B1, B2 helps the body convert carbohydrate into energy.

Vitamin B2 aids in the formulation of growth hormones, a primary factor in muscle health and development. It also contributes to healthy red blood cell production. Red blood cells are the carriers of oxygen to working muscles, making them an integral part of performance
Best sources: legumes, pseudograins, nuts, brown rice, nutritional yeast, and blackstrap molasses.

Vitamin B3

Vitamin B3 is essential for the body's breakdown and utilization of carbo-hydrate and protein. As with other B vitamins, vitamin B3 plays an integral part in the conversion of food into energy. Vitamin B3 has an important role in keeping the digestive system healthy as well. A healthy digestive system will allow the body to get more out of its food, reducing hunger and the amount of food needed. Also, a healthy digestive system will extract trace minerals from food, essential for performance.
Best sources: beets, sunflower seeds, nutritional yeast.

Vitamin B5

As with other B vitamins, vitamin B5 helps the body convert food into energy. As well, vitamin B5 facilitates the production of steroids—an integral part of the regeneration process after exertion. This vitamin is found in a wide variety of healthy foods, and deficiency is uncommon.
Best sources: seeds, pseudograins, avocados.

Vitamin B6

As a B vitamin, B6 too participates in the release of energy from food and in the formation of red blood cells. Vitamin B6 aids in the production of antibodies—essential for warding off infection and maintaining the ability to recover from exertion quickly. Vitamin B6 contributes to cardiovascular health, helping the heart efficiently circulate blood in a greater volume as demanded by the active person.
Best sources: pseudograins, greens, bananas, brown rice, walnuts, avocados, oats.

Folate (Folic Acid)

Folate is a B vitamin that is found naturally in foods; when in supplement form, it is called folic acid. Folate works in tandem with vitamin B12 to help produce oxygen-carrying red blood cells. Folate plays an integral role in helping the body make use of dietary protein, facilitating muscle repair. The heart relies on folate, in part, to help it maintain a smooth, rhythmic, efficient beat—and gives it a higher tolerance for physical activity.
Best sources: leafy green vegetables, legumes, pseudograins, orange juice, nutritional yeast.

Vitamin B12

Vitamin B12 is essential for a healthy nervous system, aiding in coordination and smooth muscle movement. As with other B vitamins, B12 plays a role in the production of red blood cells and conversion of food to usable energy. Unlike other B vitamins, B12 is not plentiful in foods. Special attention must be paid to ensure dietary B12 needs are met, particularly if the diet doesn't contain animal products and exercise level is moderate to high.
Best sources: chlorella, miso, nutritional yeast, kombucha.

Vitamin C

Vitamin C is a powerful antioxidant, meaning it plays an integral role in reducing damage to body tissue and muscle done by physical activity; it is therefore essential for active people. Cellular damage that occurs as a result of environmental factors, such as pollution, will be minimized by daily ingestion of vitamin C. The ability to minimize environmental stress will greatly improve the body's ability to ward off infection and allow it to recover from physical activity considerably quicker. Iron absorption is improved when iron is ingested at the same time as vitamin C–rich foods. Best sources: most vegetables and fruits (especially citrus fruits).

Vitamin D

Vitamin D allows the body to absorb calcium more efficiently—a key factor for proper bone formation (and healing) and smooth muscle contractions. Best sources: nutritional yeast, exposure to sunlight.

Vitamin E

Vitamin E, like vitamin C, is a powerful antioxidant. Active people need higher levels of vitamin E than sedentary people, as vitamin E, in concert with other vitamins, reduces the constant stress exercise places on the body.

Promoting cardiovascular health by maintaining an optimal ratio of "good" to "bad" cholesterol is another role of vitamin E. The ability to maintain the ideal ratio is a key factor for proper growth hormone production—the cornerstone of muscle rejuvenation post-exertion. Vitamin E also combats the effects of harmful free radicals produced by physical activity. Best sources: flaxseed oil, hemp oil, pumpkin seed oils, and especially raspberry seed, cranberry seed, and pomegranate seed oils; nuts, avocados.

Vitamin K

Vitamin K plays a significant role in blood clotting. It also provides the heart with nutrients it needs for optimal function.
Best sources: leafy green vegetables, pine nuts.

Biotin

Biotin works in concert with the B vitamins as a converter of food into usable energy.

It is also necessary for cell growth and helps the production of fatty acids and the metabolism of fats and amino acids.

Best sources: nuts, nutritional yeast.

Carotenoids

Carotenoids are fat-soluble phytochemicals, meaning that they are stored in fat cells and not excreted in urine. Therefore, they remain in the body longer. A class that includes over 600 naturally occurring pigments synthesized by plants, algae, and photosynthetic bacteria, carotenoids are easily spotted since they are yellow, orange, deep green, and red. Many of them also have antioxidant properties and include

- Alpha-carotene
- Beta-carotene
- Cryptoxanthin
- Lutein
- Lycopene
- Zeaxanthin

Best sources: carrots, sweet potatoes, squash, spinach, kale, collard greens, tomatoes, red and yellow sweet peppers. Most colorful fruits and vegetables.

MACROMINERALS

Calcium

For most people, bone strength and repair is calcium's major role. Active people, however, have another important job for the mineral: muscle contraction and ensuring a rhythmic heartbeat. Upward of 95 percent of the body's calcium is stored in the skeleton, and a decline in calcium levels may take years to manifest as osteoporosis. But a decline will be noticeable as an irregular heartbeat and muscle cramps—the responsibilities of that remaining few percent. Since calcium in the bloodstream is lost in sweat and muscle contractions, a higher dietary level for active people is recommended.

The body orchestrates the effective combination of calcium and vitamin D to maximize calcium absorption.

Best sources: leafy green vegetables, unhulled sesame seeds, tahini.

Magnesium

Critical for muscle function, magnesium helps the heart beat rhythmically by allowing it to relax between beats, which allows all other muscles to relax. Magnesium also assists in calcium's bone production.

Best sources: leafy green vegetables, string beans, legumes, pseudograins, bananas, nuts, avocados.

Phosphorus

Critical in the maintenance of the body's metabolic system, phosphorus allows the body to use food as fuel. Phosphorus works with calcium in the production, repair, and maintenance of bones.

Best sources: pseudograins, most tropical fruit.

Potassium

Potassium, an electrolyte, helps the body maintain fluid balance and therefore hydration. Being properly hydrated is essential for efficient movement. Proper hydration will maintain the blood's light viscous flow, increasing the amount the heart can pump and improving performance. Smooth, concise muscle contractions are one of potassium's responsibilities. Nerve impulse transmission and cell integrity also rely, to a degree, on potassium. As a result, smooth motor function, heartbeat efficiency, and the ability to strongly contract a muscle are dependent on adequate potassium intake. As with other electrolytes, potassium is lost in sweat, so active people need more.

Best sources: leafy green vegetables, most fruits (especially bananas and kiwis).

Sodium

Sodium is a vital component of nerves as it stimulates muscle contraction and helps to keep calcium and other minerals soluble in the blood. With too little, muscle stiffness and cramping can be the result.

TRACE MINERALS

Boron

Important for bone health and strength, boron has also been linked to a reduction in free radical production during the conversion of food into usable energy. Deficiency may result in reduced motor skills and difficult learning. Best sources: fruits, vegetables, nuts and legumes.

Chloride

Vital in the production of hydrochloric acid, chloride is secreted from the parietal cells of the stomach in preparation for digestion
Best sources: sea vegetables, sea salt.

Chromium

Chromium works with other vitamins and minerals to turn carbohydrate into usable energy.
Best sources: pseudograins, nuts, nutritional yeast, black pepper, thyme.

Cobalt

A component of vitamin B12, cobalt is a nutritional factor necessary for the formation of red blood cells.
Best sources: chlorella, miso, nutritional yeast, kombucha.

Copper

Like vitamin C, copper assists iron absorption in the body. With iron, copper plays a role in the transport of oxygen throughout the body— imperative for optimal performance. As a member of the body's defense

network, copper works in concert with antioxidants to reduce the effects of environmental and physical damage, providing the body with a strong platform to regenerate and build strength.
Best sources: legumes, seeds, pseudograins, raisins, nuts.

Iodine

Iodine is integral to thyroid hormone production. Thyroid hormone assists the cells in the fabrication of protein and the metabolism of fats—essential for energy maintenance. High levels of iodine are lost in sweat, making active people's requirements higher than those of less active people.
Best sources: sea vegetables (especially dulse).

Iron

The main role of iron is to fabricate hemoglobin to facilitate red blood cell health. An adequate iron level is of paramount importance for the active person. A well-maintained iron level ensures the body is able to deliver oxygen-rich blood to the hard-working extremities, maximizing efficacy. Also used to build blood proteins needed for food metabolism, digestion, and circulation, dietary iron is essential for proper functionality.
Best sources: spinach, legumes (especially split peas), pumpkin seeds.

Manganese

As an activator of antioxidant enzymes, manganese contributes to an expedited process of recovery, essential to all those who are physically active. Manganese is a cofactor in energy production, metabolizing protein and fats.
Best sources: leafy green vegetables, legumes, pseudograins, nuts, rice.

Molybdenum

A trace mineral, molybdenum's chief role is as a mobilizer, moving stored iron from the liver into the bloodstream—of particular significance to active people. An aid in the detoxification processes, molybdenum helps the body rid itself of potentially toxic material, minimizing stress.
Best sources: legumes, pseudograins, nuts.

Selenium

In concert with vitamin E, selenium preserves muscle tissue elasticity, allowing fluent, supple movement. A trace mineral, selenium combines with other antioxidants to shield red blood cells from damage done by physical exertion. It also improves immune function. As with other antioxidants, selenium offers protection from environmental stress encountered by most people on a regular basis.
Best sources: Brazil nuts, walnuts, whole-grain rice, nutritional yeast.

Zinc

Zinc's major role is to allow the body to use dietary protein as building blocks, for the regeneration of muscles. As well, zinc plays an integral role in the preservation of proper immune function.
Best sources: pseudograins, pumpkin seeds, nutritional yeast.

MY FAVORITE RESTAURANTS AND CAFÉS

BEETS LIVING FOODS CAFÉ (Austin)

5th Street Commons
1611 W 5th Street, Suite 165
Austin, TX 78703
www.beetscafe.com

Beets Living Foods Café features an upscale raw-food dining experience. Owner/Operator Sylvia Heisey is passionate about healthful living and sharing it with the world; the chefs of Beets Café create uncommonly good food that is alive with flavor and nutrition and prepared with love. The menu utilizes seasonal vegetables, fruits, nuts and seeds, and the chefs' first choice is always local and organic, supporting farmers with sustainable practices that preserve the Earth. Meal selections, packaged in eco-friendly containers, are also available for take-out.

BLOSSOMING LOTUS (Portland)

1713 Northeast 15th Avenue
Portland, OR 97212
(503) 228-0048
www.blpdx.com

Located in the historical Irvington district on Portland's East Side, Blossoming Lotus is open seven days a week to provide customers with a wide array of organic, vegan, sustainable meals.

CANDLE 79 (New York City)

154 East 79th Street at Lexington Avenue
New York, NY 10021
(212) 537-7179
www.candle79.com

Candle 79 is the upscale, elegant sister restaurant of the famous Candle Café, whose famed vegan, organic cuisine is presented in a different setting:

a two-floor fine dining oasis with an organic wine and sake bar for the conscientious yet sophisticated eater. Candle 79 has twice been rated as Zagat's #1 vegetarian restaurant, and its reputation is known internationally. It is the restaurant choice of neighborhood regulars, celebrities, politicians, and corporate tycoons.

Combining creative, beautifully presented healthy, and delicious cuisine with gracious and knowledgeable service in a gorgeous duplex space, Candle 79 is at the forefront of a movement to bring elegance to vegetarian cuisine, and to bring the concepts of "local," "seasonal," "organic," and "vegan" into the culinary mainstream.

CRU (Los Angeles)

1521 Griffith Park Blvd
Los Angeles, CA 90026
(323) 667-1551
www.crusilverlake.com

In the Silverlake area of Los Angeles, Cru serves up delicious, seasonal, organic, raw food that is nutrient-rich and perfectly flavor-balanced.

CRUDESSENCE (Montreal)

105 Rachel Street West
Montreal, QC H2W 1G4
(514) 510-9299
www.crudessence.com

A healthy oasis in the heart of the city, Crudessence serves vegan, organic, and local living food in an inspired atmosphere. The Crudessence team emphasizes respect for all living things: a healthy body in a clean environment and a strong, sustainable ecosystem. A full range of catering services and an accompanying culinary academy are integral parts of Crudessence's mandate to instill in others the happiness of conscious eating and support for local agriculture.

FRESH AT HOME (Toronto)

www.freshrestaurants.ca

Fresh on Bloor

326 Bloor Street West
Toronto, ON M5S 1W5
(416) 531-2635

Fresh on Crawford

894 Queen Street West
Toronto, ON M6J 1G3
(416) 913-2720

Fresh on Spadina

147 Spadina Avenue
Toronto, ON M5V 2L7
(416) 599-4442

With a comprehensive menu, and three locations, Fresh offers a wide variety of nutrient-dense healthy fast food for eat in or take away. Also, their menu of fresh juices is impressive.

GORILLA FOOD (Vancouver)

101-436 Richards Street
Vancouver, BC V6B 2Z3
(604) 684-3663
www.gorillafood.com

Started by an organic, vegan, raw food enthusiast, Gorilla Food is passionate about creatively and consciously providing raw, organic, vegan foods to people who care for themselves and the world. Gorilla's kitchen and eat-in space is at 436 Richards Street in the bustling core of downtown Vancouver. It also provides a line of vegan raw food ingredients, available at select retail environments. Finally, Gorilla's convenient delivery service brings the best locally sourced raw foods directly to the customer, connecting the urban consumer with organic farmers who are growing natural foods in the most sustainable ways.

THE GREEN DOOR (Ottawa)

198 Main Street
Ottawa, ON K1S 1C6
(613) 234-9597
www.thegreendoor.ca

Since 1988, the daily practice in the kitchen and bakery of The Green Door Restaurant reflects a desire to create delicious and wholesome food that is as close to its natural state as possible. Recipes are kept simple; there are no fillers, processed ingredients, or preservatives in any of the dishes. There is no set menu; every morning, the team assesses the day's supply of fresh vegetables, and creates the menu based on what ingredients are in season or in plentiful supply—although some popular dishes are produced daily. The Green Door specializes in high-quality foods made from ingredients that are locally produced.

HORIZONS (Philadelphia)

611 South 7th Street
Philadelphia, PA 19147-2103
(215) 923-6117
www.horizonsphiladelphia.com

Over the years, Horizons has become a major contributor to the dining scene in Philadelphia. In 2006, Horizons was awarded "3 Bells" by *Philadelphia Inquirer* restaurant critic Craig LaBan. That same year, it was named "Restaurant of the Year" by *VegNews* magazine. Since then, Horizons continues to be celebrated on a local and national level as one of the pioneers of vegan cooking. Horizons has been recognized by *Philadelphia Magazine* as one of the Top 50 Restaurants in Philadelphia and by the *New York Times* as one of Philadelphia's Best New Restaurants. Horizons made culinary history on November 4, 2009, by cooking the first vegan dinner at the prestigious James Beard House in New York City.

JIVAMUKTEA CAFÉ (New York City)

2nd Floor, 841 Broadway
New York, NY 10003
(800) 295-6814
www.jivamuktiyoga.com/cafe/index.html

Located within Jivamukti Yoga School, JivamukTea Café's mission is to facilitate the elevation of consciousness and support the practice of ahimsa (non-harming) through delicious, nourishing, vegan meals that use organic foods free from genetic modification and by employing sustainable practices that support the continued viability of all precious life forms on our shared planet. It provides a peaceful and educational environment for all to enjoy food, drink, art, music, and community events that support and expand upon this vision.

KARYN'S ON GREEN (Chicago)

130 South Green Street
Chicago, IL 60607-2625
(312) 226-6155
www.karynsongreen.com

With delicious food and a vibrant bar scene, Karyn's on Green is making vegan sexy in the midst of Chicago's traditional Greektown neighborhood. It serves lunch, dinner, and drinks seven days a week in a chic atmosphere, providing an earth-friendly vegan approach to contemporary dining. The diverse menu features classic American dishes reinterpreted with innovative presentations but without the meat, fish, chicken, or dairy—and highlights a host of satisfyingly bold flavors and imaginative combinations.

KARYN'S FRESH CORNER CAFÉ (Chicago)

1901 North Halsted Street
Chicago, IL 60614
(312) 255-1590
www.karynraw.com/Raw-Cafe

Karyn's Fresh Corner Café is a one-of-a-kind holistic wellness center. Founder Karyn Calabrese is committed to using only whole fresh foods (organic) whenever possible. Fresh Corner creates fresh, delicious, high-quality meals that are high in fiber and low in fat. Consistency is the key to making healthy lifestyle choices, and the Café's Living Food Menu helps consumers maintain that consistency. The Café also features classes and workshops throughout the year on the importance of food choices and how to prepare tasty, nutritious meals at home.

LIFE FOOD GOURMET (Miami)

1248 SW 22nd Street
Miami, FL 33145-2936
(305) 856-6767
www.lifefoodgourmet.com

Life Food Gourmet offers fresh and creative raw meals and snacks, from simple to extravagant.

LIVE ORGANIC FOOD BAR (Toronto)

264 Dupont Street
Toronto, ON M5R 1V7
(416) 515-2002
www.livefoodbar.com

Live is proud to offer an array of gourmet, gluten- and sugar-free vegan dishes to invigorate and cleanse the body, mind, and soul. Many different cultural foods and ingredients are combined in handmade organic dishes. Each dish is prepared and served by experienced staff and guided by Live's founders, internationally known Raw Chef and restaurateur Jennifer Italiano and her financial partner and brother, restaurateur Chris Italiano. With their deep love of food and service, they ensure a life-changing culinary experience.

MILLENNIUM (San Francisco)

580 Geary Street
San Francisco, CA 94102-1650
(415) 345-3900
www.millenniumrestaurant.com

Millennium creates a gourmet dining experience out of vegetarian, healthy, and environmentally friendly foods, striving to make vegetarian dining fun and exciting. Nestled in the heart of a food lovers' city, Millennium is committed to keeping that tradition alive. The cuisine is influenced by the flavors and styles of many cultures and all dishes are completely animal-free. Millennium is dedicated to supporting the essential earthly concepts of organic food production: small farms, sustainable agriculture, recycling, and composting. The kitchen cooks with fresh produce delivered every day, and chooses organic whenever possible; the restaurant is completely free of genetically modified foods.

PURE FOOD & WINE (New York City)

54 Irving Place
New York, NY 10003
(212) 477-1010
www.oneluckyduck.com/purefoodandwine

Even though I haven't used any recipes from Pure Food & Wine in this book, I want to mention and highly recommend this restaurant. It's gourmet raw food at its finest. My friend Sarma (who has also written a couple of excellent books, *Raw Food/Real World* and *Living Raw Food*) is the founder and chef.

RAVENS' RESTAURANT (Mendocino)

44850 Comptche Ukiah Road
Mendocino, CA 95460-9007
(707) 937-5615
www.ravensrestaurant.com

Located at Stanford Inn Eco-Resort on the Mendocino coast, Ravens' Restaurant is haute contemporary vegetarian and vegan cuisine blended with ecologically responsible paradigms. Dishes are based on locally harvested products from seaweed to morels; 99 percent of all ingredients are organic, and most produce is from regional organic growers or the Inn's California-Certified Organic Farm. The wine list comprises primarily wines produced from certified organic vineyards, biodynamic vineyards, or those using sustainable, traditional farming practices. All food wastes are composted and the compost dug back into garden beds; all glass, papers, and cardboard are sent to recycling. Ravens' Restaurant is independently owned and lovingly cared for by Jeff and Joan Stanford.

THRIVE JUICE BAR (Waterloo)

105-191 King Street South
Waterloo, ON N2J 1R1
(519) 208-8808
www.thrivejuicebar.com

Named after my first book *Thrive*, Thrive Juice Bar was started by a big supporter of the plant-based whole food philosophy that I put forth in my book. Now a friend, founder Jonnie serves up some of the best-tasting, most nutrient-dense smoothies you'll ever drink.

CALCULATING THE NUMBERS

CHAPTER 2   EATING RESOURCES

The Greatest Emission Creator

Since a midsize car emits ½ pound of CO_2 to travel 1 mile (www.falconsolution.com/co2-emission/), we can calculate the following:

CANADIAN BEEF EMISSIONS

256 km (distance needed to drive a mid-size car to produce the equivalent in CO_2e as the production of 1 kg of beef) × 31.1 kg (average annual beef consumption of each Canadian) = 7961 km. converted to miles: 4976

4976 × 33,311,400 (Canadian population) = 166,757,526,400 miles ÷ 238,857 miles (average distance to the moon) = 693,961 trips to the moon

Driving distance from Vancouver to Toronto: 2719 miles (4375 km)

U.S. BEEF EMISSIONS

256 km (distance needed to drive a midsize car to produce the equivalent in CO_2e as the production of 1 kg of beef) × 43.8 kg (average annual beef consumption of each American) = 11,278 km. converted to miles: 7008

7008 × 307,006,550 (U.S. population) = 2,151,501,902,400 miles ÷ 238,857 miles (average distance to the moon) = 9,007,489 trips to the moon

CANADIAN CHICKEN EMISSIONS

23.5 km (distance needed to drive a midsize car to produce the equivalent in CO_2e as the production of 1 kg of chicken) × 30 kg (average annual chicken consumption of each Canadian) = 703 km (439.4 miles)

U.S. CHICKEN EMISSIONS

23.5 km (distance needed to drive a mid-size car to produce the equivalent in CO_2e as the production of 1 kg of chicken) × 46.5 kg (average annual chicken consumption of each American) = 1086 km (679 miles)

CANADIAN PORK EMISSIONS

Since for every 1 kg of pork produced, 5 kg of CO_2 is released, that's the same amount of CO_2e as driving 18.25 miles.

29.3 km (distance needed to drive a midsize car to produce the equivalent in CO_2e as the production of 1 kg of pork) × 22.9 kg (average annual pork consumption of each Canadian) = 672 km (418 miles)

U.S. PORK EMISSIONS

29.3 km (distance needed to drive a midsize car to produce the equivalent in CO_2e as the production of 1 kg of pork) × 29.6 kg (average annual pork consumption of each American) = 867 km (538 miles)

What Constitutes Environmentally Friendly Food Choices?

1335 miles conserved × U.S. population = 409,853,744,250 miles ÷ 238,857 miles average distance to the moon = 1,715,895.98 trips to the moon

For the light breakfast: emission savings would be 26% (light is 10 ÷ 38 of traditional). Therefore, savings from eating the plant-based option over the "light" option would conserve as much CO_2 as would be emitted by driving the equivalent distance as making 446,133 trips to the moon.

CHAPTER 3   AN APPETITE FOR CHANGE

Nutrient-to-Emission Ratio

Formula: CO_2e, in grams, emitted in the production of 1 kg of given food divided by the number of calories per 1 kg of given food. The nutrient density of the given food divided by the quotient of the above calculation yields the nutrient-to-emission ratio.

$$\frac{CO_2e, \text{ in grams, emitted in the production of 1 kg of food}}{\text{number of calories per 1kg of food}} = \begin{array}{l} CO_2e, \text{ in grams,} \\ \text{emitted to produce} \\ 1 \text{ calorie of food} \end{array}$$

$$\frac{\text{nutrient density of the food}}{CO_2e, \text{ in grams, emitted to produce 1 calorie of food}} = \text{nutrient-to-emission ratio}$$

Since the eatlowcarbon.org suggested serving size is 4 oz (¼ pound), you can find the amount of CO_2e that is emitted in the production of 1 kg of each food by multiplying the amount of CO_2e emitted by 4 oz by 4, which will give you the amount of CO_2e emitted by one pound of the food. To convert that to 1 kg, multiply by 2.2.

You can use Nutri-Facts.com to find out how many calories are in each 100 g of that food and then multiply that number by 10 to give you the amount in 1 kg.

Here's an example using beef:

7641 g of CO_2e per 4oz.* 7641 × 4 (to yield amount of CO_2e for 1 lb) = 30,564 × 2.2 (to convert to 1 kg) = 67,240 ÷ 3410 (calories per 1 kg[†]) = 19.7 grams of CO_2e needed to produce 1 calorie from beef. 20 (nutrient density of beef[‡]) ÷ 19.7 = 1.02.

Beef tenderloin steak has a nutrient-to-emissions ratio of 1.02.

* eatlowcarbon.org
[†] Nutri-Facts.com
[‡] eatrightamerica.com/nutritarian-lifestyle/Measuring-the-Nutrient-Density-of-your-Food

ALMONDS
20 × 4 = 80 × 2.2 = 176 ÷ 5810 = 0.03. 38 ÷ 0.03 = 1266
Almonds have a nutrient-to-emissions ratio of 1266.

LENTILS
56 × 4 = 224 × 2.2 = 492.8 ÷ 1160 = 0.42. 100 (nutrient density) ÷ 0.42 = 238.
Lentils have a nutrient-to-emissions ratio of 238.

STEAMED VEGETABLES
83 × 4 = 332 × 2.2 = 730.4 ÷ 650 = 1.1. 300 ÷ 1.1 = 272
Steamed vegetables (combo of carrots, broccoli, asparagus) have a nutrient-to-emissions ratio of 272.

FRESH WILD LOCAL COHO SALMON

$101 \times 4 = 404 \times 2.2 = 888.8 \div 1390 = 0.64. \ 39 \div 0.64 = 61$

Fresh wild local coho salmon has a nutrient-to-emissions ratio of 61.

BAKED CHICKEN BREAST

$436 \times 4 = 1744 \times 2.2 = 3836 \div 1650 = 2.32. \ 27 \div 2.32 = 11.6$

Baked chicken breast has a nutrient-to-emissions ratio of 11.6.

POACHED EGGS

$661 \times 4 = 2644 \times 2.2 = 5816 \div 1420 = 4.01. \ 27 \div 4.01 = 6.7$

Poached eggs have a nutrient-to-emissions ratio of 6.7.

FARMED FRESH SALMON

$1203 \times 4 = 4812 \times 2.2 = 10,585 \div 1780 = 5.9. \ 39 \div 5.9 = 6.6$

Farmed fresh salmon has a nutrient-to-emissions ratio of 6.6.

DOMESTIC CHEDDAR CHEESE

$1140 \times 4 = 4560 \times 2.2 = 10,032 \div 4030 = 2.49. \ 10 \div 2.49 = 4$

Domestic cheddar cheese has a nutrient-to-emissions ratio of 4.

BEEF TENDERLOIN STEAK

3410 calories per 1000 g.

7641 in CO_2e per 4 oz = 7641×4 (lbs) $\times 2.2$ (converting to kg) = 67,240 ÷ 3410 (calories per 1 kg) = 19.7 grams of CO_2e needed to produce 1 calorie from beef. 20 (nutrient density) ÷ 19.7 = 1.02.

Nutrient density: 20

Beef tenderloin steak has a nutrient-to-emissions ratio of 1.02.

Nutrient-to-Arable-Land Ratio

Formula: By weight, amount of plant food divided by animal food that can be grown on an equal amount of land. Multiply that number by how many times greater in nutrient density the plant food is over the animal food. Take that number and divide it by how many times greater in calorie density the animal food is over the plant food. (Occasionally, the plant food will be more calorie dense, in which case you'll multiply those two numbers.) This will tell you how much more land (in multiples) will be needed to produce, calorie for calorie, the equivalent in micronutrient content for the two foods that you compared.

Please note that in "Calculating the Numbers," I've rounded to two decimal places. Inconsequential discrepancies in calculations will occur if you round to more or fewer decimal places in your calculations.

CATTLE FEED VERSUS BEEF

Since it takes 16 pounds of cattle feed to yield 1 pound of beef,* we can determine how much land would be needed to yield the equivalent micronutrient level from cattle feed itself, compared to beef.

Looking at a traditional cattle feed makeup (half corn and the other half composed of half wheat and half soybeans), we get a nutrient density of 41.25.

Since beef has a nutrient density of 20, I divided 41.25 by 20 to get the difference in nutrient density.

41.25 ÷ 20 * = 2.06 (difference in nutrient density)

Multiplying the 16 (multiple of how much more cattle feed is needed than beef to produce the same weight of food) × 2.06 (difference in micronutrient level between cattle feed and beef) = 33. That means that 33 times more land would need to be used to gain the equivalent micronutrient levels from beef as from wheat/corn/soybeans.

To compare calories to calories (as opposed to weight to weight), we can find out the amount of calories in 1 kg of each of the foods, then find the difference. I use Nutri-Facts.com to do this.

Since beef has 1.41 times more calories than an equal weight of wheat, corn, and soy† (in the combination mentioned: ½ corn, ¼ soybeans, and ¼ wheat), we can divide 33 (times more land needed to gain micronutrients from beef as opposed to an equivalent weight of cattle feed) by the amount that beef is more calorie dense than cattle feed, which is 1.41. That equals

23.4. Therefore, calorie for calorie, we'd need 23.4 times more land to gain the same amount of nutrition from beef as compared to the nutrition we'd gain from the food we fed to the cow.

*using eatrightamerica.com
† using nutritional data from Nutri-Facts.com

16 (multiple of cattle feed, by weight, that is fed to a cow as opposed as to what is returned in food) × 2.06 (nutrient density of cattle feed, 41.25, divided by nutrient density of beef, 20) = 16 × 2.06 = 33 (32.96 rounded).

33 ÷ 1.41 (times more calorie dense beef is than cattle feed is) = 23.4

HEMP VERSUS BEEF

880 (pounds of hemp grown per acre) divided by 165 (pounds of beef produced on an acre) = 5.33 × 3.25 (how many times more nutrient dense hemp is than beef) = 17.33 × 3 (times by which hemp is more calorie dense than beef) = 51.9

KALE VERSUS BEEF

38,400 (pounds of kale grown per acre) divided by 165 (pounds of beef produced on an acre) = 232 × 50 (how many times by which kale is more nutrient dense than beef) = 11,600 divided by 4 (times by which beef is more calorie dense than kale) = 2900

Nutrient-to-Water Ratio

SWEET POTATOES VERSUS BEEF

Formula: Difference in nutrient density (in multiples) × difference in amount of water (in multiples) required to produce each crop on the same amount of land. Divide that number by the number of multiples the animal food is more calorie dense than the plant food is (if not more dense, then multiply those two numbers).
Nutrient density of beef: 20
Nutrient density of sweet potatoes: 83

Amount of water required to produce 1 pound of beef: 2500 gallons (minimum)

Amount of water required to produce 1 pound of sweet potatoes: 60 gallons

Beef has 3.3 more calories than sweet potatoes for an equal weight (900 calories per 1 kg of sweet potato compared with 2990 calories per 1 kg of beef)

$83 \div 20 = 4.15 \times 41.66$ ($2500 \div 60$, difference in amount of water required, in multiples) $= 172.88 \div 3.3 = 52.3$

Nutrient to Fossil Fuel Comparison

LENTILS VERSUS ANIMAL PROTEIN

25.29 average nutrient density of animal products

26.9 average number of calories of energy required to produce 1 calorie of protein from animals

2.2 number of calories of energy required to produce 1 calorie of protein from lentils

100: nutrient density of lentils

Nutrient-to-Emission Comparison

Difference in CO_2e (in multiples) that it takes to produce an equal weight of the two foods, divided by the multiple by which animal food is more calorie dense than plant food. (Occasionally, the plant food will be more calorie dense, in which case you'll multiply the two numbers.) Take that number and multiply it by the difference (in multiples) that the plant food is more nutrient dense.

Here's an example:

LENTILS VERSUS CHICKEN

CO_2e

Lentils: 1 lb = 224 g CO_2 emission equivalent. $224 \div 2.2$ (to kg) $= 101.82$

Baked chicken: 1 lb = 1744 g CO_2 emission equivalent. $1744 \div 2.2 = 792.73$

$792.73 \div 101.82 = 7.79$

7.79 times more CO_2e is released into the atmosphere to produce the same amount (in weight) of chicken as lentils.

To calories:

1160 cal per 1 kg lentils

1650 cal per 1 kg chicken breast

$1650 \div 1160 = 1.4$ more calories for equal weight of chicken

$7.8 \div 1.4 = 5.57$ times CO_2 equivalent calorie to calorie

Nutrient density of lentils = 100

Chicken = 27

3.7 times more nutrient dense × 5.57

3.7×5.57 times CO_2 equivalent calorie to calorie = 20.6

STEAMED VEGETABLES VERSUS BAKED SALMON

Calorie to calorie:

Steamed vegetables (cauliflower, carrots, broccoli): 1 lb = 333 g CO_2e

Baked farmed coho salmon: 1 lb = 4812 g CO_2e

$4812 \div 333 = 14.45$ times more CO_2 will be released into the atmosphere to produce an equal weight of coho salmon compared to steamed vegetables

1780 calories per 1 kg of coho salmon

650 calories per 1 kg of cauliflower, carrots, broccoli

$1780 \div 650 = 2.74$

Average nutrient density of cauliflower, carrots, broccoli = 304

Nutrient density of salmon = 39

$304 \div 39 = 7.8$ times more nutrient dense

$14.45 \div 2.74 = 5.27 \times 7.8 = 41.44$

NUTS VERSUS DOMESTIC CHEESE

Calorie to calorie:

Raw nuts: 1 lb = 80 g CO_2e

American cheese: 1 lb = 4560 g CO_2e

$4560 \div 80 = 57$ times CO_2e

5810 cal per 1 kg (equal combination of raw almonds, cashews, walnuts, and pistachios)

4030 cal per 1 kg American cheese

$5810 \div 4030 = 1.44$

Average nutrient density of nuts (almonds, cashews, walnuts, pistachios)
= 36.75
American cheese = 10
36.75 ÷ 10 = 3.7 times more nutrient dense nuts are than American cheese
57 × 1.44 = 82.02 × 3.7 = 304

KIDNEY BEANS VERSUS BEEF TENDERLOIN

Calorie to calorie:
Beef tenderloin: 1 lb = 30,564 g CO_2e
Beans: 1 lb = 96 g CO_2e
30,564 ÷ 96 = 318.37 times more CO_2e is released into the atmosphere to produce the equivalent in weight of beef as of kidney beans

Nutrient density:
Nutrient density of kidney beans = 100
Nutrient density of beef = 20
100 ÷ 20 = 5

Conversion to calories from weight:
Since there are 2.69 times more calories in 1 kg of beef than there are in kidney beans, to compare calories to calories, we divide by 2.69
1270 calories per 1 kg
3410 calories per 1 kg
3410 ÷ 1270 = 2.69
318.38 × 5 = 1591.85 ÷ 2.69 = 591.76
Pound for pound:
Beef tenderloin: 1 lb = 30,564 g CO_2e
Beans: 1 lb = 96 g CO_2e
30,564 ÷ 96 = 318.37 times more CO_2e is released into the atmosphere to produce the equivalent in weight of kidney beans and beef

Nutrient density of kidney beans = 100
Nutrient density of beef = 20
100 ÷ 20 = 5
318.37 × 5 = 1591

The Low Cost of High Nutrition

Black beans to eggs:
Black beans: 1320 cal per 1 kg
Eggs: 1430 cal per 1 kg
1430 ÷ 1320 = 1.08
Black beans cost per pound: $1.59
Eggs cost per dozen: $3.99
Eggs cost per pound (9 eggs): $2.99
12 ÷ 9 = 1.33
3.99 (cost of 12 eggs) ÷ 1.33 = 3.98 (close to 3.99, cost of 12 eggs)
2.99 ÷ 1.59 = 1.88
To gain calories from black beans would cost 1.88 times less than to get them from eggs
Black beans nutrient density: 83
Eggs nutrient density: 27
83 ÷ 27 = 3.07
1.88 ÷ 1.08 = 1.74 × 3.07 = 5.37

Lentils to chicken:
Lentils: 1060 cal per 1 kg
Chicken: 1650 cal per 1 kg
1650 ÷ 1060 = 1.55
Lentils cost per lb: $1.99
Chicken cost per pound: $4.99
$4.99 ÷ $1.99 = 2.5
Lentils nutrient density: 100
Chicken nutrient density: 27
100 ÷ 27 = 3.7
65 ÷ 39 = 1.66
2.5 ÷ 1.55 = 1.6 × 3.7 = 5.96

Flaxseed to salmon:
Flaxseed: 5340 cal per 1 kg
Salmon: 1900 cal per 1 kg
5340 ÷ 1900 = 2.8

Flaxseed cost per pound: $1.79
Salmon cost per pound: $15.99
15.99 ÷ 1.79 = 8.9
Flaxseed nutrient density: 65
Salmon nutrient density: 39
65 ÷ 39 = 1.66
2.8 × 8.9 × 1.66 = 41.37

For more details on the calculations in this section, you may visit www.brendanbrazier.com.

NOTES

1 Health's Dependence on Nutrition

1. Centers for Disease Control and Prevention, *Stress ... at Work, DHHS (NIOSH) Publication Number 99–101* (National Institute of Occupational Safety and Health [NIOSH], 1999), NIOSH Publications and Products webpage, www.cdc.gov/niosh/docs/99-101/.

2. WGBH Educational Foundation and the Harvard Medical School Division of Sleep Medicine, "Why Sleep Matters: Benefits of Sleep," Healthy Sleep Web Site, http://healthysleep.med.harvard.edu/healthy/matters/benefits-of-sleep.

3. C. Gronfier, R. Luthringer, M. Follenius, N. Schaltenbrand, J.P. Macher, A. Muzet, G. Brandenberger, "A Quantitative Evaluation of the Relationships Between Growth Hormone Secretion and Delta Wave Electroencephalographic Activity During Normal Sleep and After Enrichment in Delta Waves," *Sleep* 19, no. 10 (1996): 817–24, www.journalsleep.org/Articles/191010.pdf.

4. World Health Organization (WHO), "Nutrition Topics: Micronutrients," WHO website, www.who.int/nutrition/topics/micronutrients/en.

5. U.S. Department of Health and Human Services (HHS) and U.S. Department of Agriculture (USDA), "Chapter 2: Adequate Nutrients Within Calories Needs," in *Dietary Guidelines for Americans 2005,* updated July 9, 2008, USDA webpage, www.health.gov/dietaryguidelines/dga2005/document/html/chapter2.htm.

6. Joel Fuhrman. Website, eatrightamerica.com/nutritarian-lifestyle/Measuring-the-Nutrient-Density-of-your-Food. See also Fuhrman, *Eat to Live: The Amazing Nutrient-Rich Program for Fast and Sustained Weight Loss,* Rev. edn. (Little, Brown, 2011).

7. Sarah Burns, "Nutritional Value of Fruits, Veggies Is Dwindling; Chemicals That Speed Growth May Impair Ability to Absorb Soil's Nutrients," *Prevention*, updated July 9, 2010, www.msnbc.msn.com/id/37396355.

8. University of Maryland Medical Center, "Omega-6 Fatty Acids" (2006), www.umm.edu/altmed/articles/omega-6-000317.htm.

9. Arthur C. Guyton, M.D., and John E. Hall, M.D., *Textbook of Medical Physiology,* Ninth edn. (W.B. Saunders, 1996), 963.

10. Ibid.

11. Diana Schwarzbein, M.D., *The Schwarzbein Principle II, The Transition* (Health Communications, Inc., 2002), 114.

12. J.C. Waterlow, "Enzyme Changes in Malnutrition," *Journal of Clinical Pathology* 4 (1970): 75–79, www.ncbi.nlm.nih.gov/pmc/articles/ PMC1176288.

2   Eating Resources: The Environmental Toll of Food Production

1. Preston Sullivan, *Sustainable Soil Management: Soil System Guide*, publication (Fayetteville, AR: National Sustainable Agricultural Information Service, National Center for Appropriate Technology, May 2004), http://attra.ncat.org/attra-pub/PDF/soilmgmt.pdf.

2. Mary Carter, "Heart Disease Still the Most Likely Reason You'll Die," CNN, November 1, 2006, www.cnn.com/2006/HEALTH/10/30/heart.overview/ index.html; "About the American Heart Association ...," Fiscal Year 2005–06, South Carolina, Fact Sheet, American Heart Association, www. americanheart.org/downloadable/heart/11453667380862005-2006%20 SC%20Fact%20Sheet.doc.

3. World Health Organization "Noncommunicable Disease Prevention and Health Promotion, Global Strategy, Facts Related to Chronic Disease, Fact Sheet," 2003, www.who.int/hpr/gs.fs.chronic.disease.shtml#:%20 WHY%20IS%20THIS%20HAPPENING?

4. "Linus Pauling—Biography," Nobelprize.org, January 26, 2011, http:// nobelprize.org/nobel_prizes/chemistry/laureates/1954/pauling-bio.html.

5. PhysicalNutrient.net, "Soil Mineral Depletion: Can a Healthy Diet Be Sufficient in Today's World?" www.physicalnutrition.net/soil-mineral-depletion.htm.

6. Organic-world.net, "Table: World: Organic Agriculture by Country: Organic Agricultural Land, Share of Total Agricultural Land, Producers 2008," www.organic-world.net/statistics-world-area-producers.html.

7. Brian Halweil, *Critical Issue Report: Still No Free Lunch: Nutrient Levels in U.S. Food Supply Eroded by Pursuit of High Yields* (The Organic Center, September 2007), www.organic-center.org/reportfiles/Yield_Nutrient_ Density_Final.pdf.

8. *Livestock's Long Shadow: Environmental Issues and Options* (Food and Agriculture Organization of the United Nations, Rome, 2006), www.fao. org/docrep/010/a0701e/a0701e00.htm.

9. Ibid.

10. R.I. Levy and J. Moskowitz, "Cardiovascular Research: Decades of Progress, A Decade of Promise," *Science* 217 (1982): 121–29.

11. Mark Gold, *The Global Benefits of Eating Less Meat: A Report by Compassion in World Farming Trust*, Foreword by Jonathon Porritt (Hampshire, UK: CWF Trust, 2004), 22, http://awellfedworld.org/PDF/CIWF%20Eat%20 Less%20Meat.pdf.

12. D. Pimentel, "Livestock Production and Energy Use," in R. Matsumura, ed., *Encyclopedia of Energy* (San Diego, CA: Elsevier, 2004): 671–76.

13. U.S. Department of Agriculture, *Agricultural Statistics* (Washington, DC: U.S. Department of Agriculture, 2001).

14. David Pimentel and Marcia Pimentel, "Sustainability of Meat-based and Plant-based Diets and the Environment," *American Journal of Clinical Nutrition* 78 (September 2003): 660S–663S, www.ajcn.org/cgi/content/ full/78/3/660S#top.

15. Hillary Mayell, "UN Highlights World Water Crisis," National Geographic News, June 5, 2003, http://news.nationalgeographic.com/ news/2003/06/0605_030605_watercrisis.html.

16. *Livestock's Long Shadow*.

17. Ibid.

18. John Robbins, "2,500 Gallons All Wet?" EarthSave Foundation website, www.earthsave.org/environment/water.htm.

19. Cornell Science News, "End Irrigation Subsidies and Reward Conservation, Cornell Water-Resources Study Advises ...," Cornell University, Ithaca, NY, January 20, 1997, www.news.cornell.edu/releases/ Jan97/water.hrs.html.

20. Cornell Science News, "U.S. Could Feed 800 Million People with Grain that Livestock Eat, Cornell Ecologist Advises Animal Scientists; Future Water and Energy Shortages Predicted to Change Face of American Agriculture," Cornell University, Ithaca, NY, August 7, 1997, www.news. cornell.edu/releases/aug97/livestock.hrs.html.

21. Anndrea Hermann, M.Sc., P.Ag- V.P. Canadian Hemp Trade Alliance 2010, email interview by author, July 28, 2010.

22. U.S. Department of Energy, "Fossil Fuels," www.energy.gov/energysources/ fossilfuels.htm.

23. GlobalPost.com, "Top 7 Suppliers of Oil to the U.S.," July 28, 2010, www.globalpost.com/dispatch/100726/top-7-us-oil-importers.

24. "The Oil Drum: Net Energy. Discussion About Oil and Our Future," www.theoildrum.com/node/3839.

25. *Petropolis: Aerial Perspectives on the Alberta Tar Sands: A Film by Peter Mettler*, dir. Peter Mettler (Greenpeace Canada), www.petropolis-film.com/#/tarsands.

26. "Peak Oil," Wikipedia.org, http://en.wikipedia.org/wiki/Peak_oil.

27. Jerome R. Corsi, "Discovery Backs Theory Not 'Fossil Fuel,'" WorldNetDaily, posted February 1, 2008, www.wnd.com/?pageId=45838.

28. United States Environmental Protection Agency, *Latest Findings on National Air Quality, 2001 Status and Trends,* EPA Publication No. EPA 454/K-02-001 (Research Triangle Park, North Carolina: U.S. Environmental Protection Agency Office of Air Quality Planning and Standards Emissions, Monitoring, and Analysis Division, 2002), www.epa.gov/air/airtrends/aqtrnd01/summary.pdf.

29. Cornell Science News, "U.S. Could Feed 800 Million People ..."

30. Ibid.

31. Ibid.

32. Food and Agriculture Organization of the United Nations, Agriculture and Consumer Protection Department, "Spotlight: Livestock Impacts on the Environment," November 2006, www.fao.org/ag/magazine/0612sp1.htm. Full report: *Livestock's Long Shadow* (see n. 820).

33. *Livestock's Long Shadow* (see n. 820), xxi.

34. Ibid.

35. *Latest Findings on National Air Quality, 2001 Status and Trends*.

36. National Institute of Environmental Health Sciences, National Institutes of Health, "Air Pollution & Cardiovascular Disease," www.niehs.nih.gov/health/impacts/cardiovascular.cfm. Full report (executive summaries and commentary): *Reanalysis of the Harvard Six Cities Study and the American Cancer Society Study of Particulate Air Pollution and Mortality: A Special Report of the Institute's Particle Epidemiology Reanalysis Project* (Health Effects Institute, 2000), http://pubs.healtheffects.org/getfile.php?u=273.

37. "Oxford Word of the Year: Locavore," OUP blog, November 12, 2007, http://blog.oup.com/2007/11/locavore.

38. Carnegie Mellon University, "Carnegie Mellon Researchers Report Dietary Choice Has Greater Impact on Climate Change Than Food Miles," News webpage, April 17, 2008, http://www.cmu.edu/news/archive/2008/April/april17_foodmiles.shtml. Full report: Christopher L. Weber and H. Scott

Matthews, "Food Miles and the Relative Climate Impacts of Food Choices in the United States," *Environmental Science & Technology* 42 (2008): 3508–13, http://pubs.acs.org/doi/pdf/10.1021/es702969f.

39. Ibid.

40. Ian Sample, "Meat Production 'Beefs Up Emissions,'" July 19, 2007, www.guardian.co.uk/environment/2007/jul/19/climatechange. climatechange. Full article: Michele Fanelli, "Meat Is Murder on the Environment," *New Scientist,* July 18, 2007, www.newscientist.com/article/ mg19526134.500.

41. Ian Sample, "Meat Production 'Beefs Up Emissions,'" July 19, 2007, www. guardian.co.uk/environment/2007/jul/19/climatechange.climatechange. Full article: Michele Fanelli, "Meat Is Murder on the Environment," *New Scientist,* July 18, 2007, www.newscientist.com/article/mg19526134.500.

42. United States Department of Agriculture, Foreign Agricultural Service, "Beef: Per Capita Consumption Summary Selected Countries, Kilograms Per Person [table]," in *Livestock and Poultry: World Markets and Trade, 2006,* www.fas.usda.gov/dlp/circular/2006/06-03LP/bpppcc.pdf.

43. Ibid.

44. "Lunar Distance: Astronomy," Wikipedia entry, http://en.wikipedia.org/ wiki/Lunar_distance_(astronomy).

45. Department for Environment Food and Rural Affairs (DEFRA), Science and Research Projects webpage, "Impacts of Food Production and Consumption—EV02007," http://randd.defra.gov.uk/Default.aspx?Menu= Menu&Module=More&Location=None&Completed=0&ProjectID=14071. Full report: C. Foster, K. Green, M. Bleda, P. Dewick, B. Evans, A. Flynn, J. Mylan, *Environmental Impacts of Food Production and Consumption: A Report to the Department for Environment, Food and Rural Affairs,* Manchester Business School (London: DEFRA, 2006), http://randd.defra.gov.uk/ Document.aspx?Document=EV02007_4601_FRP.pdf.

46. Ibid.

47. "Beef: Per Capita Consumption Summary Selected Countries ..."

48. Ibid.

49. Ibid.

50. Ibid.

51. Dominic Kennedy, "Walking to the Shops 'Damages Planet More Than Going by Car,'" *The Times*, August 4, 2007, www.timesonline.co.uk/tol/ news/science/article2195538.ece.

52. "Vega for Sustainability and Reducing Your Carbon Foot Print," http://myvega.com/sustainability. Values calculated using Falcon Solution's CO_2 Emissions Calculator (www.falconsolution.com/co2-emission).

53. Ibid.

3 An Appetite for Change: Environmental and Health Solutions Through Food

1. Department of Energy and Climate Change [U.K.], "Legislation: Climate Change Act 2008," www.decc.gov.uk/en/content/cms/legislation/cc_act_08/cc_act_08.aspx.

2. Carbon Trust, "The Carbon Reduction Label," www.carbon-label.com.

3. *Case Study CTS055: Working with Tesco: Product Carbon Footprinting in Practice* (London, UK: Carbon Trust, 2008), www.carbontrust.co.uk/publications/pages/publicationdetail.aspx?id=CTS055. www.carbon-label.com/casestudies/Tesco.pdf.

4. Whole Foods Market, "Health Starts Here" webpage, www.wholefoodsmarket.com/nutrition.

5. Anndrea Hermann, email interview (see chap. 2, n. 33).

6. Cornell Science News, "U.S. Could Feed 800 Million People ..." (see chap. 2, n. 20).

7. North Williamette Research and Extensive Center, Oregon State University, "Commercial Vegetable Production Guides: Collards and Kale," last revised April 23, 2002, http://nwrec.hort.oregonstate.edu/collards.html; Pimentel and Pimentel, "Sustainability of Meat-based and Plant-based Diets and the Environment" (see chap. 2, n. 26).

8. Values calculated using Falcon Solution's CO_2 Emissions Calculator (www.www.falconsolution.com/co2-emission). 2.837 tonnes of carbon dioxide.

9. U.S. Department of Energy, *Transportation Energy Data Book*, Edition 29 (June 30, 2010), http://cta.ornl.gov/data/index.shtml.

4 Eight Key Components of Good Nutrition

1. University of Maryland Medical Center, "Omega-3 Fatty Acids" (2006), www.umm.edu/altmed/articles/omega-3-000316.htm.

GLOSSARY

Abiogenic theory

Proponents theorize that oil is not fossil fuel but rather originates from deep carbon deposits created during the formation of the earth. Abiogenic theorists point to the discovery of methane on Saturn's moon Titan as evidence supporting the hypothesis that hydrocarbons can form without biology, and they don't believe we are in danger of running out of oil.

Aerobic exercise

Aerobic means with oxygen. Any exercise that requires the constant breathing of oxygen to maintain pace is considered aerobic. Running at a moderate pace is an aerobic form of exercise, while sprinting full-out is not. Sprinting is classified as anaerobic, that is, without oxygen.

Anthropogenic

Of, relating to, or resulting from human influence on the natural world. For example, *anthropogenic climate change* refers to changes in the climate attributed to human activity.

Antioxidants

Antioxidants are the name given to several naturally occurring compounds—vitamin C, vitamin E, selenium, and carotenoids—prized for their cell-protection and cell-regeneration attributes. They help remove body-aging and cancer-causing free radicals from the body.

Arable land

Land fit for the growing of food. It must be in a climate conducive for agriculture with soil with sufficient nutrients to sustain crops.

Biological age

Biological age refers to the time that has passed since the body's most recent round of cellular regeneration. Biological age can be reduced by speeding the regeneration process of the body. Complementary stress, such as exercise and high-quality food, reduces biological age, while uncomplementary stress and refined foods increase it.

Biological debt

Biological debt refers to the state of fatigue the body goes into after energy from stimulation has dissipated. It is often brought about by eating refined sugar or drinking coffee to gain short-term energy.

Carbon dioxide (CO$_2$)

The gas emitted from the combustion of fossil fuel, carbon dioxide is known as a greenhouse gas.

Catabolic

A metabolic state in which a "breaking down" rather than a "building up" occurs in body tissues is referred to as catabolic. This state is most commonly precipitated by stress and therefore by the release of cortisol.

Celiac disease

Celiac disease is the intolerance of gluten-containing foods, such as wheat. A celiac who consumes gluten risks damaging the small intestine.

Climate change

Generally known as an altering of weather patterns over the course of several years, the term *climate change* is most commonly used to refer to an anthropological shift in climate (one that his caused by humans). However, climate change can be used to refer to both natural and anthropological shifts in climate. Global warming is the best known form of climate change.

CO$_2$e

CO$_2$e is an internationally accepted abbreviation for carbon dioxide equivalent. It's a measure that expresses the amount of all greenhouse gases released into the atmosphere, not just carbon dioxide. Other greenhouse gases, such as methane and nitrous oxide, have a global warming potential (GWP) considerably greater than that of CO$_2$ (carbon dioxide), therefore CO$_2$e takes their potency into account to allow for comparisons to be drawn between multiple sources that emit different forms of gas.

Electrolytes

Electrolytes are electricity-conducting salts. Throughout our body tissue, fluid, and blood, electrolytes conduct charges that are essential for muscle contractions, heart beats, fluid regulation, and general nerve function. Chloride, calcium, magnesium, sodium, and potassium are the chief minerals in electrolytes. A diet too low in these minerals can cause muscle cramps and heart palpitations. When we drink too much liquid that does not contain electrolytes, it can flush out the body's remaining electrolytes, causing muscle cramping and heart palpitations.

Emissions

Emissions generally refer to gases (such as carbon dioxide) created by the burning of fossil fuel. Methane and nitrous oxide are also examples of emissions.

Empty food

This term is usually assigned to foods that are heavily processed or refined. With little if any nutritional value, such foods still have plenty of "empty" calories, and usually starch and sugar, all of which can lead to quick weight gain and a feeling that hunger is never being satisfied.

Energy independent

Achieving energy independence—the desirable state of not requiring energy (oil, for the most part) to be imported from other countries—has been a long-standing goal of the United States, for both economic and national security reasons. It's widely accepted that energy independence will not be possible until the United States dramatically reduces its demand and develops alternative forms of energy—for example, solar and wind power, and biofuels from sustainable sources such as algae—on a large scale.

Essential fatty acids (EFAs)

EFAs are fats that cannot be produced by the body but must be obtained through food in order to achieve peak health. Omega-3 and omega-6 are the two essential fatty acids.

Fractionalized

Food that is no longer whole is termed fractionalized. White flour, for example, is fractionalized, because the germ and the bran components of the wheat have been removed, leaving only the flour.

Free radicals

Free radicals are damaging compounds that alter cell membranes and can adversely affect our DNA. Occurring naturally in the body, free radicals are produced on a daily basis in small amounts. However, as stress increases, so too does the production of free radicals. If stress is allowed to persist in the body for an extended period, the damage done by free radicals can be significant; they have been linked to cancer and other serious diseases. Research has also shown that free radicals cause premature signs of aging when they remain in the system. Reducing stress through better nutrition is one way to combat free radical production. Specifically, antioxidants help rid the body of free radicals by helping it excrete them in urine and sweat.

Fructose

Also known as fruit sugar, fructose is naturally occurring in most fruits. Since it is very sweet, it is often extracted from fruits to sweeten other foods.

Genetically modified organism (GMO)

A GMO is an organism whose genetic makeup has been altered using genetic engineering techniques—usually in an effort to enable more food to be grown on less land. Genetic modification is most commonly performed on crops such as corn and soy to help them survive being sprayed with pesticides. The practice is a concern within the scientific community as well as among the general public because no long-term studies have been done to determine the safety of GMOs.

Global warming

The increase in Earth's average atmospheric and water temperature since the mid-twentieth century is known as global warming. Greenhouse gases are thought to be the prime cause.

Global warming potential (GWP)

GWP is a measure of the amount of greenhouse gas released into the atmosphere. Carbon dioxide is assigned a 1, meaning it's the benchmark against which other gases are measured. Methane, for example, is 23 times as potent as carbon dioxide in terms of its damaging environmental attributes; therefore, its GWP is 23.

Glucose

Glucose is a form of simple carbohydrate and the primary sugar found in the blood. The best Thrive source for glucose is dates.

Greenhouse effect

The trapping of the sun's warmth within the earth's atmosphere by greenhouse gases is known as the greenhouse effect. The greenhouse effect is considered to be the largest contributing factor to hastening global warming.

Greenhouse gases

Gases emitted into the atmosphere that prevent a large portion of the sun's heat from leaving the Earth's atmosphere, leading to global warming. Greenhouse gases include carbon dioxide, methane, and nitrous oxide, which are emitted from a variety of sources, including the combustion of fossil fuels and the raising of livestock for food.

Growth hormone

Growth hormone, often simply referred to as GH, is what stimulates muscular growth and cell reproduction. It is released during intense exercise and sleep.

High-net-gain nutrition

Net gain is the term I use to refer to the usable nutrition the body is left with once food is digested and assimilated. Food that is nutrient dense and requires little energy to digest and assimilate can be referred to as high-net-gain food. The higher the net gain of food, the more energy that can be garnered from it.

Lignans

Lignans are plant-derived compounds that combine with others to fabricate the cell wall of the plant. Lignans are regarded as one of the best compounds to help protect against cancer and reduce cholesterol levels. When we consume lignan-rich foods, friendly bacteria convert the plant lignans to mammalian lignans, thereby allowing the release of their therapeutic attributes within the body.

Livestock

Livestock are domesticated animals raised in an agricultural setting for the production of food. They include animals that will directly become food, as well as animals that produce food, such as milk and eggs.

Methane

A greenhouse gas, methane is released from livestock, primarily ruminants, such as cattle and sheep.

Muscular functionality

Muscles that are fit and move with ease while putting minimal strain on the cardiovascular system because of their superior efficiency can be said to have become functional. Strength equals efficiency, which culminates in muscular functionality.

Nitrous oxide

A greenhouse gas with a GWP considerably higher than methane and carbon dioxide, nitrous oxide is released from livestock waste.

Nutrient density

A ratio by which micronutrient content is averaged and divided by calories. Nutrient density is an attribute to seek when striving healthier food options.

Organic

Foods grown without the use of synthetic herbicides or pesticides are said to be organic. All food was organic until the mid-twentieth century, when new synthetic chemicals were introduced to food crops in an effort to reduce damage done by weeds, insects, and rodents. The hope at that time was that this novel way of farming would allow the production of more food on less land. But since then people have become concerned about the effects on their health of ingesting chemical residues on food. Non-organic food is often referred to as "conventional."

Peak oil theory

This theory defines "peak oil" as the point at which global oil extraction has reached its maximum rate, after which the rate of production enters "terminal decline."

Phytonutrient

Also referred to as a phytochemical, a phytonutrient is a plant compound that by boosting the immune system offers health benefits beyond its nutritional value. Classified as micronutrients, phytonutrients are not essential for life but can help improve vitality and, in turn, the quality of life. See "Guide to Nutrients" on page 293 for more information.

Ruminant

A mammal that digests plant-based food by moistening it within its first stomach, then regurgitating the semi-digested mass, "cud," and re-chewing it. This process, "ruminating," breaks down plant matter and stimulates digestion. Cows, goats, and sheep are ruminants that are commonly farmed for their meat and by-products.

Simple carbohydrate

Sometimes referred to as simple sugar, simple carbohydrate is prevalent in most fruits. The body's most readily usable form of fuel, and therefore its first choice for fuel, simple carbohydrate is necessary for both mental and physical activity. If the body is not fed foods that contain simple carbohydrate, it will have to convert complex carbohydrates, but that conversion takes extra work and therefore is not a good use of energy. Glucose and fructose, the primary simple carbohydrates, are ideal fuels in that they are already in a form that the body can utilize. As well, digestive enzymes can break these simple carbs down more efficiently than they can their complex carbohydrate counterparts.

Sterols

Sterols are steroid-like compounds found in both plants and animals. Plant sterols have the ability to lower cholesterol and have been recognized as beneficial to heart health and in the fight against cardiovascular disease.

Strength-to-weight ratio

The amount of weight able to be lifted in comparison to body weight is known as the strength-to-weight ratio. It is particularly advantageous for endurance athletes to increase this ratio, because becoming stronger will garner no performance improvement if body weight also rises. This is because the extra weight of the muscle will offset the strength gains. Strength-to-weight ratio can be increased by building muscular strength (and therefore efficiency and practical function) while not increasing the size or weight of the muscle.

Trace minerals

Also known as microminerals, trace minerals have several important functions in the body that add up to optimal health. As the name suggests, these minerals are needed only in trace amounts, and a diet rich in a variety of foods will ensure their inclusion.

Trans fats

Also known as trans-fatty acids, these are a form of fat produced by heating oils to high temperature, thus altering their chemical compound and making these fats difficult for the body to process. They also inhibit the body's ability to efficiently burn healthy fats as fuel.

Whole food

Food that has had no nutrient—macro or micro—removed during processing.

RESOURCES

BOOKS

Environment

Barlow, Maude. *Blue Covenant: The Global Water Crisis and the Coming Battle for the Right to Water*

Hartmann, Thom. *Last Hours of Ancient Sunlight: The Fate of The World and What We Can Do About It Before It's Too Late*

Heinberg, Richard. *The Party's Over: Oil, War and the Fate of Industrial Societies*

Goodall, Chris. *How to Live a Low-Carbon Life: The Individuals Guide to Tackling Climate Change*

Suzuki, David, and David Taylor. *The Big Picture: Reflections on Science, Humanity, and a Quickly Changing Planet*

Tamminen, Terry. *Cracking the Carbon Code: The Key to Sustainable Profits in the New Economy*

Health

Barnard, Neal D. *Dr. Neal Barnard's Program for Reversing Diabetes: The Scientifically Proven System for Reversing Diabetes without Drugs*

Campbell, T. Colin, and Thomas M. Campbell II. *The China Study: The Most Comprehensive Study of Nutrition Ever Conducted And the Startling Implications for Diet, Weight Loss, And Long-term Health*

Freedman, Rory, and Kim Barnouin. *Skinny Bitch*

Fuhrman, Joel. *Eat to Live: The Revolutionary Formula for Fast and Sustained Weight Loss*

Food and Recipes

Esselstyn, Rip. *The Engine 2 Diet: The Texas Firefighter's 28-Day Save-Your-Life Plan that Lowers Cholesterol and Burns Away the Pounds*

Melngailis, Sarma. *Living Raw Food: Get the Glow with More Recipes from Pure Food and Wine*

Morris, Julie. *Superfood Cuisine: Cooking with Nature's Most Amazing Foods*

Phyo, Ani. *Ani's Raw Food Essentials: Recipes & Techniques for Mastering the Art of Live Food*

Ronnen, Tal. *The Conscious Cook: Delicious Meatless Recipes That Will Change the Way You Eat*

Silverstone, Alicia. *The Kind Diet: A Simple Guide to Feeling Great, Losing Weight, and Saving the Planet*

Steele, Jae. *Ripe from Around Here: A Vegan Guide to Local and Sustainable Eating (No Matter Where You Live)*

Wignall, Judita. *Going Raw: Everything You Need to Start Your Own Raw Food Diet and Lifestyle Revolution at Home*

Food Issues

Heintzan, Andrew, and Evan Solomon (eds). *Feeding the future: From Fat to Famine, How to Solve the World's Food Crises*

Joseph, John. *Meat Is for Pussies*

Moby and Miyun Park (eds). *Gristle: From Factory Farms to Food Safety (Thinking Twice About the Meat We Eat)*

Pollan, Michael. *In Defense of Food: An Eater's Manifesto*

Schlosser, Eric. *Fast Food Nation: The Dark Side of the All-American Meal*

Weber, Karl (ed). *Food Inc.: A Participant Guide: How Industrial Food Is Making Us Sicker, Fatter, and Poorer-And What You Can Do About It*

MOVIES

Blue Gold: bluegold-worldwaterwars.com

Flow: flowthefilm.com

Forks over Knives: forksoverknives.com

Fuel: thefuelfilm.com

Future of Food: thefutureoffood.com

King Corn: kingcorn.net

Supersize Me: super-size-me.morganspurlock.com

WEBSITES

Nutrition / Environment / Recipes / Blogs / Health

The Kind Life: Alicia Silverstone's blog includes writings on health, nutrition, style, and the environment. Also includes a forum and serves as an excellent plant-based recipe archive.
thekindlife.com

Crazy Sexy Life: Includes a daily blog and article posting by a large number of leaders in the know about plant-based health, nutrition, and style. Started by Kris Carr, from the film *Crazy, Sexy, Cancer.*
crazysexylife.com

Heather Mills: Information about her ongoing projects, including charity work and her plant-based V-Bites Café and food products. Includes regularly updated health, nutrition, and fitness advice.

heathermills.org

Georges Laraque: Former NHL player and (as of September 2010) deputy leader of the Green Party of Canada. Includes video interviews and a regularly updated blog about environmental issues and training as an elite athlete while eating a plant-based diet.

georgeslaraque.com

VegNews magazine online: The home of the popular magazine includes the latest information on plant-based nutrition, restaurants, and all things related to leading a plant-based life. Includes a blog and video content.

vegnews.com

John Mackey: The blog of the founder and CEO of Whole Foods Market always contains an intelligent, proactive, and well thought out applicable message, often including articles about Conscious Capitalism, a movement created by Mackey.

www2.wholefoodsmarket.com/blogs/jmackey

Vega Community: An active forum on all things related to nutrition, health, sports, training, and the environment. Visitors may create a profile and post questions as well as gain access to the latest information on topics of interest to them.

vegacommunity.com

Elizabeth Kucinich: Sound food, environmental, and political suggestions.

ElizabethKucinich.com

Ecocentric: The official blog for sustainable food, water and energy programs of the GRACE Foundation.

ecocentricblog.org

Sustainable Table: Advocates for and celebrates local sustainable food, educates consumers on food-related issues, and works to build community through food.

sustainabletable.org

Meatless Monday: A non-profit initiative of The Monday Campaigns, in association with the Johns Hopkins Bloomberg School of Public Health. Its goal is to help you reduce your meat consumption by 15 percent in order to improve your personal health and the health of the planet.

meatlessmonday.com

The Eat Well Guide: Offers free resources, maps, and directories for finding fresh, locally grown, and sustainably produced food in the United States and Canada.

eatwellguide.org

The Meatrix films: Award-winning humorous satires (translated into more than

30 languages) that educate about the dark origins of industrial food production.
themeatrix.com

H2O Conserve: An online source for tools and information—including the popular Water Footprint Calculator—which enable individuals to make water conservation part of their everyday lives.
h2oconserve.org

Mind Body Green: Provides a wealth of information about nutrition, health, and the environment. Updated daily.
mindbodygreen.com

En*theos: Philosophical information delivered in approachable, easy to grasp language.
entheos.me

H Life Media: H Life is an online holistic-health lifestyle publication to redefine the concept of health, to inform us about what it truly means to lead a healthy lifestyle, and to empower us to take responsibility for our wellness and our lives.
hlifemedia.com

G Living: The go-to site for the modern green movement. G Living showcases all that is fresh and green in the world of food, fashion, transportation, architecture, and more.
gliving.com

Choosing Raw: A wealth of plant-based-nutrition information with near-daily updates, entertaining and informative blog posts, and recipes.
choosingraw.com

No Meat Athlete: A comprehensive blog focusing on plant-based nutrition for athletes.
nomeatathlete.com

Julie Morris: A regularly updated blog on food, health, and green living. It also includes excellent videos of plant-based recipe preparation.
juliemorris.net

Olsen Haus: A source for high-fashion, environmentally friendly shoes.
olsenhaus.com

Physicians Committee for Responsible Medicine: Doctors and laypersons working together for compassionate and effective medical practice, research, and health promotion. PCRM is a nonprofit organization.
pcrm.org

T. Colin Campbell Foundation: A non-profit organization, the TCCF offers scientific and health information available to the public, without influence from industry or commercial interests.

tcolincampbell.org

Dr. Joel Fuhrman: A wealth of information on disease prevention through nutrient-dense whole foods.
drfuhrman.com

Centers for Disease Control and Prevention: Collaborating to create the expertise, information, and tools that people and communities need to protect their health through health promotion, prevention of disease, injury and disability, and preparedness for new health threats.
cdc.gov

World Health Organization: WHO is the directing and coordinating authority for health within the United Nations system. It is responsible for providing leadership on global health matters, shaping the health research agenda, setting norms and standards, articulating evidence-based policy options, providing technical support to countries, and monitoring and assessing health trends.
who.int

Organic Athlete: A non-profit organization whose mission is "to promote health and ecological stewardship among athletes of all ages and abilities by sharing information, building community, and inspiring through athletic example."
organicathlete.org

7th Generation Advisors: Advocating environmental and clean energy policies by providing advice and guidance to visionary political leaders and emerging clean technology firms worldwide.
seventhgenerationadvisors.org

Environment / Policies

Carbon Trust: The Carbon Trust is a not-for-profit company with the mission to accelerate the move to a low carbon economy. It provides specialist support to help business and the public sector cut carbon emissions, save energy, and commercialize low carbon technologies.
carbontrust.co.uk

Carbon Reduction Label: The Carbon Reduction Label indicates the amount of CO_2 used to produce a product. The label also indicates that the company is actively working to reduce its carbon footprint.
carbon-label.com

David Suzuki Foundation: It works with government, business, and individuals to conserve our environment by providing science-based education, advocacy, and policy work, as well as acting as a catalyst for the social change that is demanded.
davidsuzuki.org

Worldwatch Institute: The Worldwatch Institute is an independent research organization recognized by opinion leaders around the world for its accessible, fact-based analysis of critical global issues. Its three main program areas include climate and energy, food and agriculture, and the green economy.
worldwatch.org

Post Carbon Institute: The Post Carbon Institute is leading the transition to a more resilient, equitable, and sustainable world through a shift away from energy derived from fossil fuel.
postcarbon.org

Department of Energy and Climate Change: The U.K.'s Department of Energy and Climate Change is responsible for all aspects of U.K. energy policy and for tackling global climate change on behalf of the nation.
decc.gov.uk

Institute for the Analysis of Global Security: IAGS is a non-profit organization that directs attention to the strong link between energy and security, and provides a stage for public debate on the various avenues to strengthen the world's energy security.
iags.org

Council on Foreign Relations: CFR is an independent, nonpartisan membership organization, think tank, and publisher.
cfr.org/about

Department for Environment Food and Rural Affairs: DEFRA is the department responsible in the U.K. government for policy and regulations on the environment, food, and rural affairs.
ww2.defra.gov.uk

New Energy Choices: Aims to promote policies that ensure safe, clean, and environmentally responsible energy options.
newenergychoices.org

United Nations: The United Nations is an international organization founded in 1945 by 51 countries and is committed to maintain international peace and security, develop friendly relations among nations, and to promote social progress, better living standards, and human rights.
un.org

Conscious Brands: A strategic planning organization that works with leaders to further expand and implement sustainability into the core of their businesses.
www.consciousbrands.com

The Ad Hatter: A search-engine optimization specialist who only takes on socially and environmentally responsible companies, specializing in nutrition sites.
theadhatter.com

Hemp History Week: A non-profit grassroots campaign that supports the legal growing of hemp for food and building materials in the United States. Advocating hemp's cultivation by presenting its health, economic, and social benefits to Congress, the backers of Hemp History Week aim to reinstate the growing of this versatile crop, thereby benefiting the American people. Hemp History Week falls in May of each year, but the group's work continues year-round.
hemphistoryweek.com

Canadian Hemp Trade Alliance: A wealth of information on everything hemp as it relates to the Canadian industry.
hemptrade.ca

Terracycle: Terracycle takes all types of garbage and turns it into consumer products with little or no waste. Upcycling, as Terracycle calls it, saves thousands of tons of garbage from going into landfills.
terracycle.net

Free Range Studios: Free Range Studios works to sell revolutionary ideas and products that build a more just and sustainable world. It is driven by a belief that the right stories told in revolutionary ways can transform society. Creators of *The Story of Stuff* and the *Meatrix*.
freerange.com

The Story of Stuff: A simple and effective 20-minute video focused on the lifecycle of consumer goods, from cradle to grave.
storyofstuff.com

Calculators

Carbon emissions from driving, air travel, and home:
terrapass.com/carbon-footprint-calculator

Water usage spanning household needs to industrial food production consumption:
www.waterfootprint.org

Automobile CO_2 based make and model:
falconsolution.com/co2-emission (used to calculate emissions in "The Great Environmental Divide: Meal Plan Comparisons" section on page 87)

Food miles:
fallsbrookcentre.ca/cgi-bin/calculate.pl

Nutritional information: Comprehensive information database that contains nutritional facts on over 6000 foods.
nutri-facts.com

Companies

Sequel Naturals: In 2003 Charles Chang (owner of his newly formed company, Sequel Naturals) and I partnered to produce a replica of the blender drink formula I had been making for myself since the early 1990s. I first began drinking it to help reduce recovery time between workouts, and it allowed me to train more and improve at a faster rate. I believe this was the defining factor that allowed me to have a career as a professional Ironman for seven years.

We launched Vega Complete Whole Food Health Optimizer in Canadian health food stores in September 2004, and the following year we began exporting it to the U.S. It's now available in most health food stores and GNCs in Canada and the U.S., and it's begun appearing in traditional supermarkets and pharmacies.

Of course, when formulating Vega products, I adhere to the nutritional and environmental ideas I write about in this book. They are nutrient-dense, high-net-gain, alkaline-forming, and plant-based, made by expending as few natural resources as possible to obtain their health boosting qualities. In fact, formulating Vega products is when I began to realize how tightly personal and environmental health was intertwined. The idea of striving to gain as many micronutrients while expending as few natural resources as possible—leading to the creation of the nutrient to resource ratio—came from my drive to develop a truly nutrient-dense, convenient, commercially available food product while limiting its strain on the environment.

The website includes recipes, informative videos, my recently published articles on health, nutrition, and environmental issues, and all things Vega.

myvega.com.

ZoN Fitness: In spring 2010, Greg Holmes of ZoN Fitness, a Chicago-based manufacturer and distributor of sporting goods, contacted me. He had read *Thrive Fitness* and felt that my approach to exercise—a tool to enhance overall quality of life—was in perfect alignment with his.

We became partners and in doing so, I created a comprehensive written and video downloadable fitness and nutrition program based on my books *Thrive* and *Thrive Fitness*. This program is free (visit zonfitness.com to access).

I was delighted to align myself with ZoN Fitness, having longed for a broad mainstream platform to disseminate what I consider to be vital information, information that I believe should be taught in school—the practical value of greater fitness and proper nutrition for long-term health. As the largest distributor of sporting goods in the world, ZoN Fitness serves as an outstanding conduit for information to an immense and diverse audience. In Canada, ZoN Fitness is available at all Canadian Tire stores, and in the United States at most sporting-goods and department stores.

Visit the website for complete information about my ZoN Fitness program, ZoN fitness equipment, and to get the latest information on health and fitness.

www.zonfitness.com.

INDEX

Also by Brendan Brazier

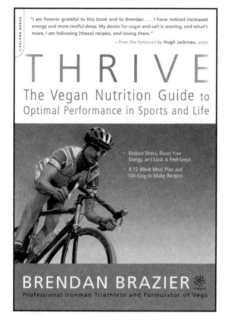

Thrive: The Vegan Nutrition Guide to Optimal Performance in Sports and Life

$14.95 | 978-0-7382-1254-8 | Paperback

Thrive features a 12-week whole foods meal plan, over 100 wheat-, gluten-, and soy-free recipes. Also includes exercise-specific recipes for pre-workout snacks, energy gels, and recovery foods.

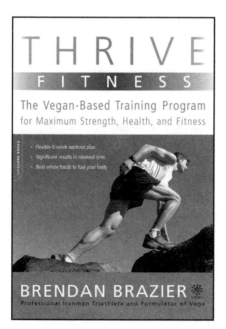

Thrive Fitness: The Vegan-Based Training Program for Maximum Strength, Health, and Fitness

$15.95 | 978-0-7382-1362-0 | Paperback

A vegan-based, performance-boosting fitness program for the busy beginner to the elite athlete. Includes:

- A complete 6-week workout plan and training log
- Illustrated exercises with step-by-step instructions
- Benefits and usage of the top 15 foods to fuel workouts
- 30 vegan, performance enhancing recipes

For more, visit **BrendanBrazier.com.**

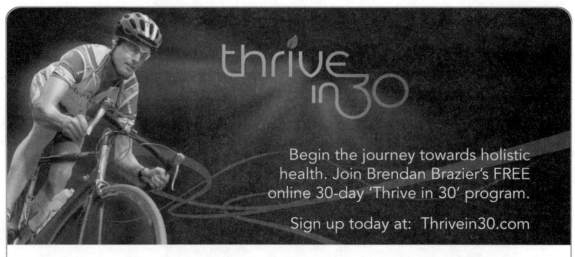

Begin the journey towards holistic health. Join Brendan Brazier's FREE online 30-day 'Thrive in 30' program.

Sign up today at: Thrivein30.com

Join Brendan Brazier as your personal guide as he walks you through the steps needed to achieve optimal performance by means of plant-based whole foods.

Based on Brendan's books (*Thrive* and *Thrive Fitness*), Thrive in 30 consists of three emails a week for four weeks, with each containing a short video and concise text component. The program is geared to help busy people seamlessly apply optimal nutritional habits and incorporate a high-return exercise program, ultimately improving their overall quality of life.

When you join Thrive in 30 you'll learn:

- How to combat stress by consuming plant-based whole foods and applying the principles of high net-gain nutrition

- Why whole food plant-based sources of protein and fat are optimal and how they can synergistically be combined with exercise to help you build a biologically younger body

- How you can alkalize your body's pH to combat disease, improve sleep quality, and shed fat

- What superfoods to eat that will balance hormones, detoxify your body, and lower cholesterol

- How to identify common foods that cause unexplained, mystery illnesses

- How to use nutrition to strategically fuel your body for greater endurance, maximize the return from workouts, and recover faster

- Why nutrition, exercise, and sleep are the secret to empowered mental health

- Strategies that will boost your health and make your gains permanent

 SIGN UP FOR FREE AT: thrivein30.com